# IntechOpen

intechopen.com

## Built by scientists, for scientists

# Meet the Authors

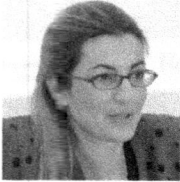

Despina Sanoudou is a Full Professor in Pharmacogenomics and Cardiovascular Biology at the Medical School of the National and Kapodistrian University of Athens, Head of the Clinical Genomics and Pharmacogenomics Unit and Co-Director of the Genetic and Pharmacogenetic Counselling Clinic at the 4th Department of Internal Medicine of the "Attikon" hospital in Athens, Greece, and CHS Associate Faculty at Harvard University. She completed her Ph.D. at the University of Cambridge, was Board-Certified in Laboratory Genetics by the American Board of Medical Genetics and Genomics, and worked as an instructor at Harvard Medical School. She has served as an expert advisor to over 25 international organizations. Her research focuses on deciphering pathogenic mechanisms in cardiovascular disease and developing precision medicine therapeutic approaches. She coordinates multiple undergraduate and postgraduate educational programs and has given lectures to thousands of students internationally. Professor Sanoudou has received numerous awards for her contributions to science and education, including the L'Oréal-UNESCO Award for Women in Science.

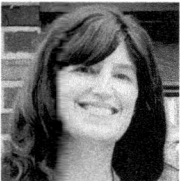

Jessica Goehringer, MS, LGC, is a senior genetic counselor with clinical expertise in multiple speciality areas, a researcher, and an associate professor in a genetic counseling graduate program. Much of her career has been focused on understanding the lived experiences of patients who undergo genetic testing for or are diagnosed with CDC tier 1 conditions (Familial Hypercholesterolemia, BRCA-related hereditary breast-ovarian cancer, and Lynch syndrome) and other genetic conditions within an internationally recognized precision medicine program. Additionally, research interest in Ehler-Danlos syndrome (EDS) led to a collaboration with the Ehlers-Danlos Society to create an app dedicated to empowering patients with EDS and providers who diagnose these conditions with the resources they need for diagnosis, management, and support.

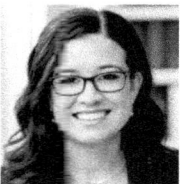

Ana Morales, MS, CGC, is an Associate Professor at the Geisinger Department of Genomic Health and a board-certified genetic counselor with over 20 years of experience. A nationally recognized expert in cardiogenetics, her work has been published in over 50 peer-reviewed publications. She co-authored the guideline for the genetic evaluation of cardiomyopathy by the Heart Failure Society of America. She served as a critical reviewer of the 2019 arrhythmogenic cardiomyopathy guideline by the Heart Rhythm Society. At Geisinger, Dr. Morales serves as the Principal Investigator of the NIH-funded IMPACT-FH grant, which promotes cascade familial hypercholesterolemia genetic testing in primary care. Her leadership includes roles in NIH ClinGen Working Groups and as the 2019 President of the American Board of Genetic Counseling.

# Contents

# Preface

In writing this book, we have drawn upon our extensive clinical and research backgrounds as geneticists and experienced genetic counselors in the fields of cardiogenetics and precision medicine. Throughout our careers, we have witnessed the exciting evolution of genetic testing technology and the understanding of the genetic contributions to cardiovascular disease. New gene-disease associations and improved variant interpretation have enabled the clinical community to harness the power of genetic testing to enhance patient care and outcomes. It has become evident that, in the era of Precision Medicine, the approach to disease diagnosis, prevention, and patient management is evolving. As such, there is a need for genetics-based care to keep pace with this development. This is especially true in the cardiovascular specialty. As genetic testing for cardiovascular disease began to be adopted in cardiology clinics over 20 years ago, the need for cardiovascular genetic counselors became apparent. This need has only intensified as professional societies, such as the American Heart Association (AHA) and the European Society of Cardiology (ESC), have published recommendations emphasizing the need for integrating genetic testing in cardiology clinics. Despite such recommendations and the availability of expanded cardiogenetic testing options, testing is underutilized. Partnering with genetic counselors who have expertise in cardiogenetics may be a solution to address this underutilization by providing expertise within a cardiovascular care delivery team that promotes more comprehensive knowledge, services, and care. Despite the well-recognized need for cardiovascular genetic counselors and the American Heart Association (AHA) recommendations to incorporate genetic counseling into cardiology practice, it remains a subspecialty of genetic counseling that does not meet the demand. Efforts are ongoing to both introduce additional genetic counselors into the workforce and to include cardiovascular-specific training for genetic counselors. During our clinical practice, we recognized the need for a comprehensive reference book that provides detailed, critical information pertinent to the cardiovascular genetic counseling process. We hope that this book will provide a comprehensive and current resource to promote the principles and practice of cardiovascular genetic counseling for a diverse audience. Students, practicing genetic counselors, clinicians, allied health professionals, and researchers may benefit from a deeper understanding of the complexities of cardiogenetics and the inherent nuances of cardiovascular genetic counselling. We hope this book provides valuable insights into the breadth of cardiovascular disease and the depth of knowledge needed to provide comprehensive cardiogenetic care. We are confident that, by becoming familiar with the contents of this book, the reader will acquire skills and develop an appreciation for the genetic counseling process, which will pave the way for improved clinical practice and ultimately enhance patient care for those affected by a personal or family history of cardiovascular disease.

**Despina Sanoudou**
Clinical Genomics and Pharmacogenomics Unit,
4th Department of Internal Medicine,
"Attikon" Hospital,
Medical School,
National and Kapodistrian University of Athens,
Athens, Greece

**Ana Morales**
Geisinger Medical Center,
Danville, PA, USA

The George Washington University,
Translational Health Sciences Program,
School of Medicine and Health Sciences,
District of Columbia, USA

**Jessica Goehringer**
Geisinger Medical Center,
Danville, PA, USA

Geisinger College of Health Sciences,
Scranton, PA, USA

## Chapter 1

# Introductory Chapter: Unraveling Inherited Cardiovascular Risk – The Role of Genetic Counseling

*Despina Sanoudou, Ana Morales and Jessica Goehringer*

## 1. Introduction

Cardiovascular diseases (CVDs) are the leading cause of death globally, representing >30% of all global deaths. While traditional cardiology has predominantly addressed the functional and structural attributes of this vital system, the burgeoning field of human genetics has progressively illuminated the profound influence of inherited variation upon cardiac development, function, and susceptibility to a diverse array of pathological states. Scientific developments have unveiled a complex architecture wherein genetic alterations exert significant modulatory effects across the spectrum of cardiovascular disease. From congenital cardiac malformations manifesting at birth to heritable cardiomyopathies that present insidiously across the lifespan, genetic variants contribute substantially to disease etiology, phenotypic expression, and therapeutic responsiveness. As the understanding of the genetic contributions to cardiovascular disease deepens, the availability of genetic testing expands. Recent recommendations by the American Heart Association, the European Society of Cardiology, the European Heart Rhythm Association (EHRA), the Heart Rhythm Society (HRS), the Asia Pacific Heart Rhythm Society (APHRS), the Latin American Heart Rhythm Society (LAHRS) and more [1–3] highlight the clinical utility of cardiovascular genetic testing. This evolving paradigm necessitates an integrated approach to cardiovascular healthcare that incorporates insights derived from the human genome to refine diagnostic precision, enhance risk prognostication, personalize therapeutic strategies, and ultimately optimize patient outcomes. The need for specialized expertise in interpreting and communicating this complex information has become paramount. This is where cardiovascular genetic counseling plays a critical role [4].

## 2. The need for genetic counselors

This specialized area of practice is dedicated to helping individuals and families understand the genetic underpinnings of heart conditions and guide patients through the complexities of genetic testing. Cardiovascular genetic counselors possess a unique skillset that encompasses not only a strong foundation in human genetics and cardiovascular disease but also specialized training in counseling techniques, risk assessment, and ethical considerations. They are adept at providing the emotional and psychosocial support necessary for the patients to cope with the implications of a genetic diagnosis, providing empathetic support and empowering individuals and families to make informed decisions aligned with their values and goals. Cardiovascular genetic counselors can therefore serve as crucial bridges, translating intricate genetic information into clinically meaningful insights.

## 3. Objectives of this book

This book is crafted to serve as an introductory guide to the principles and practice of cardiovascular genetic counseling, illuminating the profound connections between our genetic inheritance and cardiovascular disease. Within these pages, readers will embark on a journey to:

- Explore the diverse ways in which genetic variations contribute to a wide array of cardiac conditions: gaining a deeper appreciation for the heritable basis of many common and rare heart disorders.

- Demystify the realm of cardiovascular genetic testing: navigate the landscape of available types of genetic tests, understanding their methodologies, clinical applications, and the crucial factors to consider when interpreting their results.

- Comprehend the indispensable role of genetic counseling: recognize the unique expertise of cardiovascular genetic counselors in facilitating understanding, providing support, and empowering informed decision-making in the context of inherited heart disease.

- Discover the foundations of pre-test evaluation and counseling: understand the critical elements of risk assessment, family history interpretation, and ethical considerations that underpin effective pre-test counseling for cardiovascular genetic testing.

- Gain knowledge in post-test interpretation and communication: understand the skills necessary to interpret complex genetic test results accurately and communicate their implications effectively to individuals and families, guiding them toward appropriate management and surveillance strategies.

- Facilitate cascade screening and family-centered care: appreciate the importance of identifying at-risk relatives and learn how genetic information can be used to implement effective cascade screening programs, promoting proactive healthcare within families.

- Explore the horizon of genetically informed cardiovascular medicine: gain insights into the exciting future of personalized cardiovascular care, where genetic profiles may guide targeted therapies and preventive interventions.

## 4. Genetic testing and counseling in CVD

Current recommendations and approaches employed toward CVD genetic testing and screening are discussed. At the pre-test level, patient selection criteria, types of genetic tests and genes being assessed are presented, along with patient education and conserting needs. At the post-test level, various interpretation considerations and challenges are presented, valuable tools and databases are provided, and genetic test result communication strategies are discussed. Special attention is given to risk determination for family members, testing minors, as well as the psychosocial implications of CVD genetic testing and ways to support patients and their families.

The field of cardiovascular genetic counseling is dynamic and constantly evolving. Advances in genomic technologies, coupled with a growing understanding of the genetic basis of heart disease, are creating new opportunities and challenges [5–8]. The integration of genomic information into routine clinical practice is becoming increasingly feasible and, sometimes, necessary, thus paving the way for more personalized and predictive approaches to cardiovascular care.

Ongoing research focused on elucidating gene-disease associations, understanding variant pathogenicity, and developing targeted therapies will continue to shape the landscape of cardiovascular genetics and, consequently, the scope of genetic counseling. The ability to identify individuals at increased risk, refine diagnoses, and potentially offer gene-based interventions will necessitate sophisticated pre- and post-testing counseling strategies to ensure appropriate utilization and informed decision-making.

## 5. Genetic counseling for polygenic and multifactorial cardiovascular disease

Beyond well-defined monogenic cardiac disorders for which guidelines have been established (e.g., including the cardiomyopathies, arrhythmias, familial hypercholesterolemia, as well as thoracic aortic aneurysm and dissection), the influence of genetic susceptibility is increasingly acknowledged in the pathogenesis of common cardiovascular diseases, including coronary artery disease, essential hypertension, and atrial fibrillation. While these conditions are undoubtedly multifactorial, with environmental and lifestyle factors exerting considerable influence, an individual's genetic constitution can significantly modulate their overall risk profile [9]. The emergence of polygenic risk scores, which aggregate the cumulative effects of numerous common genetic variants, represents a promising avenue for refining risk stratification and potentially guiding targeted preventive interventions in these complex diseases that constitute a significant burden on global health.

## 6. Pharmacogenetic counseling

Furthermore, the discipline of pharmacogenomics, which investigates the impact of an individual's genetic makeup on their response to pharmacological agents, is gaining increasing relevance in cardiovascular therapeutics. Genetic variants can influence pharmacodynamics and pharmacokinetic parameters, impacting efficacy and safety for commonly prescribed cardiovascular medications such as anticoagulants, antiplatelet agents, and lipid-lowering therapies [10]. Meanwhile, new highly targeted biological drugs will often require genetic testing prior to administration [11, 12]. The integration of pharmacogenomic data into clinical decision-making holds the potential to optimize drug selection, tailor dosage regimens, and minimize the risk of adverse events, thereby facilitating more personalized and efficacious pharmacological management of cardiovascular disease.

In this evolving scientific milieu, the role of the cardiovascular genetic counselor will be increasingly vital. Their expertise will be essential for ensuring that individuals and families can effectively navigate the complexities of genomic medicine and benefit from its potential.

## 7. How will healthcare professionals benefit from this book

This book aspires to serve as a valuable resource for a broad spectrum of healthcare professionals seeking a deeper understanding of the genetic dimensions of cardiovascular health:

- Cardiovascular clinicians: enhance your ability to integrate genetic information into your practice, leading to more precise diagnoses and personalized management plans.

- Genetic counselors: expand your expertise in this specialized and increasingly vital area of genetic medicine.

- Primary care physicians: develop a heightened awareness of the genetic underpinnings of common cardiovascular conditions and learn when referral for genetic evaluation is indicated.

- Nurses and allied health professionals: gain a comprehensive understanding of the genetic aspects of cardiovascular care to provide more informed and supportive patient care.

- Students and researchers: acquire a robust foundation in the principles and applications of cardiovascular genetic counseling, paving the way for future contributions to this dynamic field.

By engaging with the knowledge contained within this book, one stands to acquire in depth understanding of the scientific knowledge and skills required in genetic counseling and profound appreciation for the genetic counseling experience. Timely, efficient, and effective integration of genetic counseling in cardiology clinics will contribute to more informed clinical practice, empowered patient decision-making, and improved outcomes for individuals and families navigating the complexities of heritable cardiovascular disease.

## Author details

Despina Sanoudou[1*], Ana Morales[2,3*] and Jessica Goehringer[2,4*]

1 Clinical Genomics and Pharmacogenomics Unit, 4th Department of Internal Medicine, "Attikon" Hospital, Medical School, National and Kapodistrian University of Athens, Athens, Greece

2 Geisinger, Danville, USA

3 Translational Health Sciences Program, School of Medicine and Health Sciences, The George Washington University, District of Columbia, USA

4 Geisinger College of Health Sciences, Scranton, PA, USA

*Address all correspondence to: dsanoudou@med.uoa.gr; amorales4@geisinger.edu and jgoehringer@geisinger.edu

## IntechOpen

# References

[1] EHRA et al. Corrigendum to: European heart rhythm association (EHRA)/ Heart Rhythm Society (HRS)/Asia Pacific Heart Rhythm Society (APHRS)/ Latin American Heart Rhythm Society (LAHRS) expert consensus statement on the state of genetic testing for cardiac diseases. Europace. 2022;**24**(8):1367

[2] Elliott P et al. Integration of genetic testing into diagnostic pathways for cardiomyopathies: A clinical consensus statement by the ESC council on cardiovascular genomics. European Heart Journal. 2025;**46**(4):344-353

[3] Musunuru K et al. Genetic testing for inherited cardiovascular diseases: A scientific statement from the American Heart Association. Circulation: Genomic and Precision Medicine. 2020;**13**(4):e000067

[4] Morales A, Goehringer J, Sanoudou D. Evolving cardiovascular genetic counseling needs in the era of precision medicine. Frontiers in Cardiovascular Medicine. 2023;**10**:1161029

[5] Dellefave-Castillo LM et al. Assessment of the diagnostic yield of combined cardiomyopathy and arrhythmia genetic testing. JAMA Cardiology. 2022;**7**(9):966-974

[6] James CA et al. International evidence based reappraisal of genes associated with arrhythmogenic right ventricular cardiomyopathy using the clinical genome resource framework. Circulation: Genomic and Precision Medicine. 2021;**14**(3):e003273

[7] Jordan E et al. Evidence-based assessment of genes in dilated cardiomyopathy. Circulation. 2021;**144**(1):7-19

[8] Sturm AC et al. Limited-variant screening vs comprehensive genetic testing for familial hypercholesterolemia diagnosis. JAMA Cardiology. 2021;**6**(8):902-909

[9] Stouras I et al. The challenge and importance of integrating drug-nutrient-genome interactions in personalized cardiovascular healthcare. Journal of Personalized Medicine. 2022;**12**(513):1-16

[10] Ingelman-Sundberg M, Pirmohamed M. Precision medicine in cardiovascular therapeutics: Evaluating the role of pharmacogenetic analysis prior to drug treatment. Journal of Internal Medicine. 2024;**295**(5):583-598

[11] Vafiadaki E et al. Pharma-cogenetically tailored treatments for heart disease. Current Pharmaceutical Design. 2010;**16**(20):2194-2213

[12] Valanti EK et al. Advances in biological therapies for dyslipidemias and atherosclerosis. Metabolism. 2021;**116**:154461

# Perspective Chapter: Genetic Counseling for Cardiovascular Disease – Part A – Pre-Test Approaches and Considerations

*Jessica Goehringer, Despina Sanoudou and Ana Morales*

## Abstract

Cardiogenetic testing was established 20 years ago; more recently, it began to be incorporated in routine clinical care. Key reasons include expanded knowledge of the genetic basis of cardiovascular disease, wider availability of enriched cardiogenetic testing panels, the issuance of clinical recommendations guiding cardiogenetic testing, and enhanced cardiologists' awareness. Cardiogenetic testing can be valuable at the levels of diagnosis, prognosis, treatment/ management selection, early disease risk detection, and personalized surveillance strategy. Cardiovascular disease-related genes are incorporated in genetic screening panels currently being evaluated for their potential in disease prevention at the general population level. These rapid developments are increasing the number of individuals requiring genetic counseling and personalized cardiovascular care. Advanced expertise is required to determine when genetic testing is needed, which genetic test is more appropriate, and how the patient and their family members should be prepared for the process. To reap the full benefits of cardiogenetic testing and screening, cardiology and genetics providers must collaborate effectively in the cardiology clinics' setting. This chapter focuses on cardiomyopathies, arrhythmias, familial hypercholesterolemia, and thoracic aortic aneurysm/dissection, as well as the specialized knowledge that cardiovascular genetic counselors need to serve their indispensable, multifaceted role when caring for individuals with these conditions.

**Keywords:** cardiovascular disease, genetic disease, genetic counseling, genetic testing, cardiovascular genetics, cardiogenetics, cardiogenomics, laboratory genetics, personalized medicine, precision medicine, gene panels, next generation sequencing, cardiomyopathies, arrhythmias, familial hypercholesterolemia, thoracic aortic aneurysm and dissection

IntechOpen

# 1. Introduction

## 1.1 State-of-the-art knowledge on CVD genetics

Genetic testing for cardiovascular disease plays a crucial role in managing cardio-vascular genetic conditions in affected patients and at-risk relatives [1]. If an individual's cardiac phenotype suggests a cardiovascular genetic condition, genetic testing should be recommended. If genetic testing is positive in the affected patient, genetic testing is recommended for their at-risk relatives to identify those who need cardiac surveillance.

Genetic testing for arrhythmias, including long QT syndrome (LQTS), catechol-aminergic polymorphic ventricular tachycardia (CPVT), and Brugada syndrome (BrS), and others, is recommended for individuals with a clinical diagnosis or strong suspicion of these conditions [2]. Similarly, genetic testing is recommended for genetic cardiomyopathies, namely dilated cardiomyopathy (DCM), hypertrophic cardiomyopathy (HCM), arrhythmogenic right ventricular cardiomyopathy (ARVC), and restrictive cardiomyopathy (RCM). Left ventricular cardiomyopathy (LVNC) requires additional considerations. Specifically, in the absence of other features, such as systolic dysfunction or a structural defect, genetic testing is not recommended for LVNC [3]. Key cutoff lab values for LDL cholesterol (LDLc) determine recommendations for familial hypercholesterolemia (FH) testing, which may be performed *via* lipid or genetic testing [4, 5]. Guidelines, also, recommend genetic testing for thoracic aortic aneurysm and dissection (TAAD), particularly for individuals who present with symptoms at age < 60 years or have a family history of TAAD, sudden cardiac death, or other related conditions [6].

With a growing list of guidelines and genetic testing options, resources are available to help providers keep abreast of those that are applicable to specific inherited cardiac conditions seen in their patients. The Cardiogenomic Guidelines Database is a searchable resource that is updated periodically and freely available. Another resource, the Cardiogenomic Testing Alliance, is formed from genomics companies and laboratories focused on cardiogenomic testing utilization. Their website offers information on evaluating patients, testing guidelines, and testing resources and also includes a guidelines database. Given that genetic testing guidelines vary by country or professional society/organization, it is relevant to note that the guidelines databases are searchable by journal or society, therefore allowing for country-specific guideline searches. Such resources can help genetic counselors and other providers worldwide to keep informed of current CVD knowledge and recommendations.

## 1.2 Expanding use of CVD genetic testing

In parallel with the profoundly deeper understanding of the genetic basis of CVD, powerful massive parallel sequencing technologies have enabled the development of a broad variety of genetic tests. The Genetic Testing Registry, supported by the U.S. National Library of Medicine, is a central location for voluntary submission of genetic test information by providers worldwide (although mostly populated by U.S.-based laboratories). It currently lists over 70,000 genetic tests, with >18,000 genes tested for >11,000 different conditions (https://www.ncbi.nlm.nih.gov/gtr/).

Hundreds of these tests are designed specifically for the detection of CVD-causing genetic variants. These usually involve the sequence assessment of CVD-related gene panels involving 1 to >300 genes (or even whole exome sequencing [WES] in exceptionally challenging cases), aiming to identify the pathogenic variant causing the disease. Different gene panels are available for a broad range of different cases, including instances where a variant in a specific gene is suspected, a specific diagnosis has been made (i.e., a well-defined CVD subcategory), or a complex clinical phenotype is observed. The cardiogenetic test results can facilitate a finite diagnosis, a more accurate prognosis, and informed guidance of clinical management. Importantly, they enable the identification of other family members at-risk of the same CVD through cascade testing (**Table 1**).

Emerging technologies, such as artificial intelligence (AI) driven tools and models for variant interpretation are being used by some laboratories to assist with variant interpretation. AI can help in analyzing large datasets, in pattern identification, and in making predications of the impact of specific variants on phenotype. Using AI can improve the time it takes to analyze data, offering the potential to increase lab volume [13]. Additionally, AI can improve result turnaround time, which can directly impact patient outcomes. However, while AI tools can improve the variant interpretation process, they have limitations. For example, these tools are unable to assess certain variant types while incomplete genotype or atypical phenotype matching can negatively impact the performance of AI models [13]. As such, human expertise is essential to validate clinical laboratory results.

Although cardiogenetic tests have been available for over three decades their integration into routine clinical care has greatly increased over the recent years largely because of: (i) expert consensus statements and recommendations from prominent international organizations highlighting the value of cardiogenetic testing, (ii) the decreasing cost of genetic testing, (iii) the development of a broader range of cardiogenetic tests that can better serve different needs (ranging from single gene, to small highly targeted, and up to whole exome or even whole genome sequencing (WGS)), and (iv) the increasing awareness of cardiologists about the availability and use of such tests, as well as their expanded continuing education on how to integrate test results into patient and family members' management.

Meanwhile, beyond the pursuit of single pathogenic gene variants, polygenic risk scores (PRS) for different forms of CVD are becoming available, promising to transform the way we predict, surveil, prevent, and/or manage CVD in the near future, by enabling a highly personalized approach (**Table 1**) [14, 15]. Unlike the aforementioned cardiogenetic tests which are aimed at identifying monogenic forms of CVD, PRS takes into consideration common genetic variants (i.e., present in >1% of the general population) which combined, can substantially increase CVD risk. Since PRS aggregate thousands of genetic variants, each contributing a small effect, they result in a probabilistic estimation of disease risk. This leads to heightened *interpretative ambiguity,* especially toward contextualizing this information alongside traditional risk factors. Unlike classical genetic tests, PRS lack binary outcomes and can be heavily influenced by environmental and lifestyle factors, making it difficult to define actionable thresholds. Furthermore, a major issue is the considerably difference performance of PRS across diverse populations due to the Eurocentric nature of most genomic datasets. This results in PRS that are often less accurate and potentially misleading when applied to non-European populations, thereby exacerbating health disparities. These parameters complicate genetic counseling and risk communication, posing challenges for genetic counselors, clinicians, and patients alike. On the ethical front, the use of PRS raises concerns regarding potential stigmatization, genetic determinism, and the risk of misinterpretation by patients. There is also a potential for misuse in contexts such as employment, insurance, or reproductive

| Term | Meaning |
| --- | --- |
| Cascade testing | The process of offering genetic counseling and testing to at-risk relatives of an individual who has been diagnosed with a genetic condition [8]. |
| Polygenic risk score (PRS) | An estimate of an individual's genetic liability to a trait or disease, calculated according to their genotype profile and relevant genome-wide association study (GWAS) data. |
| Variant of unknown significance (VUS) | Genetic variants with uncertain association to pathological conditions. These variants have contradicting pathogenic and benign evidence or are so rare in the general population that little information is available about them. |
| Actionable findings | Actionable findings generally refer to genetic findings that enable medically beneficial actions for the patient. However, as it gives little indication of the scope, quality, or availability of the action, it may be used to convey variable concepts [9]. |
| Mutation | A mutation is defined as a permanent change in the nucleotide sequence [10]. |
| Polymorphism | A common variant in a specific sequence of DNA. "Common" is typically defined as an allele frequency of at least 1% in the general population [10]. |
| Genetic variants | Genetic variants are differences in DNA sequence that occur naturally between individuals in a given population. Because the terms "mutation" and "polymorphism", often lead to confusion due to incorrect assumptions of pathogenic and benign effects respectively, it is recommended that both terms be replaced by the term "variant" with the following modifiers: [1] pathogenic (P), [2] likely pathogenic (LP), [3] uncertain significance (VUS), [4] likely benign (LB), or [5] benign (B) [10]. |
| Autosomal dominant | Inheritance pattern involving a genetic variant that is located on an autosome (chromosomes 1–22), and has a dominant effect (i.e., only one copy of it suffices to cause the condition). |
| Autosomal recessive | Inheritance pattern involving a genetic variant that is located on an autosome (chromosome 1–22), and two copies of it are required to cause the condition. |
| X-linked | Inheritance pattern involving variants in genes on the X chromosome, |
| Variable expressivity | Variable expressivity refers to the range of signs and symptoms (from mild to severe) that can occur in different people with the same genetic condition. |
| Reduced (incomplete) penetrance | Penetrance refers to the proportion of people with a particular genetic variant who exhibit signs and symptoms of a genetic disorder. If some people with the variant do not develop features of the disorder, the condition is said to have reduced (or incomplete) penetrance [7]. |
| Incidental findings (IFs) or Unsolicited findings (UFs) | Genetic findings that have medical relevance but are not related to the indication for testing and not intentionally sought during analysis [11]. |
| Secondary findings (SFs) | Genetic findings are not related to the indication for testing, but they are identified as a result of a deliberate search for medically relevant variants [12]. |

**Table 1.**
*Glossary (the basic concepts relating to the terms of the glossary are elaborately explained in Ref. [7]).*

decision-making, highlighting the need for robust regulatory frameworks. Informed consent becomes particularly complex, as patients must understand the nuanced nature of risk conveyed by PRS, along with its limitations and potential downstream implications. Addressing these challenges will require interdisciplinary collaboration to develop standards for accuracy, clinical utility, and ethical guidelines to ensure that the use of PRS enhances rather than complicates patient care.

The increasing number of genetic testing tools, their broadening clinical applications and value are driving increased demand, and consequently leading to a rapidly growing healthcare systems' need for specialized cardiogenetic counseling experts.

## 1.3 Genetic population screening for cardiovascular disease

Historically, genetic testing for the disease was phenotype or family history-driven. However, the transformative advances in genomic analysis, coupled with lower testing costs and a focus on precision medicine make population screening possible [12, 16, 17]. An estimated 1.2–3.5% of the population has a highly penetrant, medically actionable pathogenic (P)/likely pathogenic (LP) variant [12, 17]. This offers the potential for early identification of individuals at increased risk, timely guideline-directed surveillance and/or pre-emptive actions for prevention, as well as earlier identification of symptoms for optimal management.

Despite the opportunity that population screening can offer, a broad range of factors need to be carefully weighted before it can be introduced in routine practice. These include feasibility, potential benefits and harms, clinical utility, health outcomes, and associated costs [18]. As such, the Genomics and Population Health Action Collaborative (GPHAC) Population Screening working group was formed in 2017. They developed a list of optimal genes to include in population screening programs and adopted the United States Centers for Disease Control and Prevention Office of Genomics and Precision Public Health's groupings of (1) Tier 1 genes: those with strong potential to improve public health on the basis of evidence-based guidelines, recommendations, and proven preventive interventions (including three genes associated with familial hypercholesterolemia), (2) Tier 2 genes: those with some evidence for medical actionability, but not ready for routine population screening, and (3) Tier 3 genes: those with limited evidence for possible medical actionability and candidates for further research [18, 19]. A 2023 study in the United States found that population genomic screening using CDC Tier 1 conditions is likely cost-effective in adults (in the United States) who are younger than 40 when testing costs is low and preventive interventions are available, while the other tiers are still under evaluation [20].

Across the Atlantic, the Council of Europe addressed the issue of population screening in the Protocol to the Oviedo Convention in 2008. It proposes factors to be considered when implementing a population screening program and is considered an international treaty, currently binding five countries and serving as a reference for other countries across Europe [21–23].

There is growing interest worldwide in population screening programs by both the general population and healthcare institutions to promote the early detection and prevention of disease and enhance wellness. With as much as 90% of the population being unaware that they have a CDC Tier 1 P/LP variant, there is ample opportunity for population screening programs to make a dramatic impact [24]. Existing programs in the United States have substantial consent rates ranging from 28% to 93%, likely indicating that the public wants access to actionable genomic information [25–27]. Over 12 programs across the U.S. are already offering genomic screening for a variety of genes (including Tier 1 genes, ACMG SF genes, or even WES and WGS) in unselected populations [18, 28].

The largest healthcare system-based population screening program in the United States is located at Geisinger Health System (GHS). In 2007, GHS initiated the MyCode® Community Health Initiative, a health-system-wide biobank that can be used broadly across the Geisinger research institute. This represents one of the earliest programs to return clinically actionable genetic results to patient participants [12, 26, 29]. Geisinger currently returns clinically actionable results (P/LP variants) for a total of 81 genes. These include the ACMG SF v2.0 genes list, in addition to genes reviewed for appropriateness and actionability. Of note, a substantial number of the genes on the ACMG secondary findings list are associated with a cardiovascular phenotype (**Table 2**).

At the time of this writing, over 350,000 participants have consented to participate in MyCode® and over 5000 results have been returned (1379448 MyCode Scorecard Update Sep24 (geisinger.org) Accessed on 9/24/2024). Among them, 87% of patient participants were not aware of their Tier 1 variant status prior to population screening [31]. Over 40% of results returned have been related to cardiovascular disease or syndromes with possible cardiovascular involvement (**Table 3**).

Similarly, 90% of individuals with Tier 1 conditions in the Healthy Nevada Project were unidentified prior to population screening [24]. This is in line with

| Phenotype | Gene(s) |
|---|---|
| Ehlers-Danlos syndrome, vascular type | *COL3A1* |
| Aortopathies (Marfan syndrome, Loeys-Dietz syndromes, familial thoracic aortic aneurysms, and dissections) | *FBN1, TGFBR1, TGFBR2, SMAD3, ACTA2, MYH11* |
| Hypertrophic and dilated cardiomyopathies | *MYBPC3, MYH7, TNNT2, TNNI3, TPM1, MYL3, ACTC1, PRKAG2, GLA, MYL2, LMNA, FLNC, TTN, BAG3, DES, RBM20, TNNC1* |
| Catecholaminergic polymorphic ventricular tachycardia | *RYR2, CASQ2, TRDN* |
| Arrhythmogenic right ventricular cardiomyopathy | *PKP2, DSP, DSC2, TMEM43, DSG2* |
| Long QT syndrome types 1–3 and 14–16, Brugada syndrome | *KCNQ1, KCNH2, SCN5A, CALM1, CALM2, CALM3* |
| Familial hypercholesterolemia | *LDLR, APOB, PCSK9* |

**Table 2.**
*ACMG SF v3.2 genes associated with cardiovascular phenotypes recommended for clinical sequencing secondary findings result return [30].*

| Condition | Results returned to patients per condition |
|---|---|
| Cardiomyopathies | 1031 |
| Familial hypercholesterolemia | 590 |
| Arrhythmias | 375 |
| Hereditary transthyretin amyloidosis | 163 |
| Heritable thoracic aortic disease | 46 |
| Marfan syndrome | 27 |
| Vascular Ehlers-Danlos syndrome | 14 |
| Loeys-Dietz syndrome | 10 |
| **Total** | **2256** |

**Table 3.**
*Summary of results returned through Geisinger's MyCode for cardiovascular disease or syndromes involving a cardiovascular phenotype as of September 1, 2024.*

the knowledge that, worldwide, an estimated 90% of individuals with FH go undiagnosed and thus without effective management [32–34].

The frequency with which population screening programs are returning actionable results that are cardiovascular in nature speaks to the importance of considering their inclusion within other population screening programs. It could allow for a personalized approach to medical care for a substantial number of patients by offering pre-symptomatic testing (e.g., electrocardiogram (ECG), lipid panel) and imaging (e.g., echocardiogram), or potentially an explanation for existing symptoms. Of course, this necessitates that the appropriate infrastructure be in place such as the availability of genetic counseling and cardiovascular care for patients with a clinically relevant result.

While population screening programs hold promise, there are implications of population-wide genetic screening to take account of. First, socioeconomic status, educational level, gender, sexual orientation, racial and ethnic diversity, and geographic location impact the uptake of population screening. Therefore, individuals from different populations may benefit more than others from population screening [35]. As institutions consider implementing population screening, they should examine whether their focus is on improving personalized care or on enhancing public health (or both), and clearly communicate this. They should also ensure the screening is equitably available and relevant to diverse populations. Individuals who agree to population screening should go through an informed consent process to make sure they have considered and understand the benefits, limitations, risks, and purpose of screening. It is especially important that they understand that population screening that does not result in an identified variant does not rule out the possibility of genetic disease. Patients should also understand what types of results are returned (e.g., what genes are included and what levels of pathogenicity) and whether pathogenicity reclassifications may be returned in the future. As with any genetic testing, it is important to understand the potential impact of receiving genetic information on the individual and family, which can increase anxiety and worry. Informed consent should include a discussion on the privacy of genetic data and what precautions are taken to uphold confidentiality. Last, we must also ethically consider what impact population screening may have on genetic discrimination. America and countries in Europe, Asia, and Oceania have taken more action in enacting laws to protect against discrimination, while many other countries have not prioritized such laws [36, 37]. Still, so, discrimination laws are not all-encompassing. For example, the U.S. Genetic Information Nondiscrimination Act (GINA) protects against health insurance and employment discrimination in cases where there are 15 or more employees but does not cover life, long-term care, or disability insurance [37]. As population screening programs continue to be introduced, efforts are needed to understand any downstream ramifications.

In summary, genetic testing for CVD is essential in identifying genetic conditions in patients and at-risk relatives, particularly for arrhythmias, cardiomyopathies, FH, and TAAD. Recent advancements, including large-scale parallel sequencing and artificial intelligence, have expanded the scope and accessibility of genetic testing and are aiding clinicians in making diagnoses. Population genetic screening is emerging as a tool for early detection of individuals who may be unaware of their increased risk of genetic disease, though it requires careful consideration of feasibility, equity, and ethical concerns. Resources like the Cardiogenomic Guidelines Database help providers stay updated on testing guidelines. While genetic testing for CVD is paramount to informing personalized care, challenges such as accessibility and proper utilization need to be addressed to ensure equitable implementation.

## 2. Incorporating genetic testing into routine clinical care requires advanced/specialized genetic counseling expertise

### 2.1 Determining if genetic testing is needed

The first step toward integrating cardiogenetic testing into routine clinical care involves expertise in determining those cases where genetic testing is needed. This involves careful consideration of pathological characteristics that could be indicative of a genetic basis for the observed phenotype. These characteristics differ among CVD. **Table 4** outlines key features suggestive of genetic cardiomyopathies, arrhythmias, familial hypercholesterolemia, and aortopathies that may warrant a genetic evaluation.

#### *2.1.1 Genetics-informed management of affected individuals*

In addition to informing surveillance in at-risk relatives, genetic testing can impact disease management in the affected patient, a stance endorsed by the American Heart Association (AHA) [1]. Antiarrhythmic therapy selection, extracardiac disease risk management, and clinical trial opportunities are relevant to affected individuals with positive genetic testing results. Selected examples are presented.

#### *2.1.1.1 Arrhythmia*

A molecular diagnosis of LQTS can inform lifestyle and therapeutic recommendations, including implantable defibrillator (ICD) placement. Similarly, in individuals with BrS, the identification of a molecular diagnosis in *SCN5A* indicates the need for aggressive arrhythmia control in those with syncope, including integration of genetic test results in the selection of defibrillator type. On the other hand, while a molecular diagnosis of CPVT is a contraindication for ICD therapy, a molecular diagnosis can inform the onset of arrhythmia susceptibility [2].

#### *2.1.1.2 Cardiomyopathy*

A diagnosis of arrhythmogenic cardiomyopathy caused by *DES*, *DSP*, *FLNC*, *LMNA*, or *PLN* variants warrants consideration of an ICD instead of a pacemaker. Additionally, the risk of sudden cardiac death and the need for heart transplantation is increased in individuals with DCM and a molecular diagnosis in *LMNA*, *DES*, *DSP*, or *RBM20*. Furthermore, some individuals with a genetic predisposition to cardiomyopathy can present with cardiac conduction disease, sinus node disease, or atrial fibrillation. These rhythm abnormalities may progress to cardiomyopathy when caused by variants in *LMNA* and *TTN* and warrant cardiomyopathy surveillance through imaging in addition to rhythm monitoring. A molecular diagnosis can also open opportunities for experimental treatments [1, 2, 38].

#### *2.1.1.3 Familial hypercholesterolemia*

Genetic testing for FH aids in clarifying the diagnosis, distinguishing it from other causes of high cholesterol, and identifying individuals with two FH-causing variants, also known as homozygous FH (HoFH). Therefore, a genetic diagnosis also aids in treatment selection, as it indicates apheresis for HoFH. Genetic testing also helps

| Condition | Key findings | | | |
| --- | --- | --- | --- | --- |
| | Imaging (echocardiogram or MRI) | Rhythm (ECG, Holter, SAECG) | Other tests, procedures | History and symptoms |
| *Cardiomyopathies* | | | | |
| DCM [38] | 95th percentile (height- and gender-based approach, per EF < 50% [39] | N/A | No CAD on LV catheterization (<50% occlusion) | Acquired causes ruled out (HIV, Chagas disease, hypothyroidism, pheochromocytoma, severe nutritional deficiency; uncontrolled hypertension, BMI >35, sarcoidosis, amyloidosis) |
| HCM [40] | LVH (IVSd >1.5 cm, LVPWd >1.5 cm) | N/A | N/A | Other causes ruled out (uncontrolled hypertension, athletic remodeling, aortic stenosis, fetal exposure to maternal diabetes) |
| ACM/ARVC* [41] | RV akinesia, dyskinesia, aneurysm, dyssynchronous RV contraction, PLAX/PSAX RVOTO, fractional area change ≤33%, increased ratio of RV end-diastolic volume to BSA, RVEF ≤40% | Inverted T waves, Epsilon waves, late potential by SAECG in at least one of the following parameters: fQRSD, LAS40, RMS40, NSVT, >500 ventricular extrasystoles [42] | RV angiography: regional RV akinesia, dyskinesia, or aneurysm Endomyocardial biopsy or autopsy: residual myocytes with fibrous replacement of the RV-free wall myocardium with or without fatty replacement | ARVC in a first degree relative, proband molecular diagnosis |
| RCM [43, 44] | Atrial enlargement, myocardial stiffness, diastolic dysfunction | N/A | N/A | Absence of amyloidosis, hemochromatosis, and other secondary causes |
| LVNC [3] | Hypertrabeculations | N/A | N/A | Conduction system disease, congenital heart defect, reduced EF |
| *Arrhythmia* | | | | |
| LQTS [45] | N/A | QTc >460 ms (men), >450 ms (women) | N/A | Syncope, seizures, SIDS, hearing loss, and syndromic features in some types. No acquired causes (heart muscle damage, electrolyte imbalance, drugs) |

| Condition | Key findings | | | |
|---|---|---|---|---|
| | Imaging (echocardiogram or MRI) | Rhythm (ECG, Holter, SAECG) | Other tests, procedures | History and symptoms |
| CPVT [46] | N/A | N/A | Exercise stress test: bidirectional VT, VA<br>Epinephrin provocation test: bidirectional or polymorphic VT | N/A |
| BrS [47] | | ST elevation in leads V1-V3, coved ST segment, ST with saddleback | | Recurrent syncope, VF, self-terminating polymorphic ventricular tachycardia, cardiac arrest, family history of SCD |
| *Hyperlipidemia* | | | | |
| FH [5] | N/A | N/A | One affected relative or unavailable family history: ≥190 mg/dL (adults); Negative family history: LDLc ≥250 mg/dL (adults) | CAD, heart attack, stroke, elevated LDL, xanthomas, xanthelasma, arcus cornealis |
| *Aortic disease* | | | | |
| TAAD [48] | Aortic aneurysm [49, 50] or dissection, mitral valve prolapses or regurgitation | N/A | N/A | N/A |

*Abbreviations: ARVC, arrhythmogenic right ventricular cardiomyopathy; BMI, body mass index; BrS, Brugada syndrome; BSA, body surface area; CAD, coronary artery disease; CPVT, catecholaminergic polymorphic ventricular tachycardia; FH, familial hypercholesterolemia; ECG, electrocardiogram; EF, ejection fraction; DCM, dilated cardiomyopathy; fQRSD, filtered QRS Duration; HCM, hypertrophic cardiomyopathy; HIV, human immunodeficiency virus; IVSd, interventricular septal thicknes in end-diastole; LAS40, low amplitude signal duration; LDLc, low density lipoprotein cholesterol; LQTS, long QT syndrome; LV, left ventricle; LVH, left ventricular hypertrophy; LVNC, left ventricular non compaction cardiomyopathy; LVPW4, left ventricular posterior wall thickness in end-diastole; NSVT, non-sustained ventricular tachycardia; PLAX, parasternal long axis view; PSAX, parasternal short axis view of the heart; QTc, QT interval, corrected; RCM, restrictive cardiomyopathy; RMS40, root mean square voltage of the last 40 ms of the QRS; RV, right ventricle; RVOTO, right ventricular outflow tract obstruction; SAECG, signal averaged ECG; SIDS, sudden infant death syndrome; TAAD, thoracic aortic aneurysm/dissection; VA, ventricular arrhythmia; VF, ventricular fibrillation; VT, ventricular tachycardia.*
*\*The findings presented herein are a summary of both major and minor criteria. A diagnosis of ARVC requires a specific combination of major and minor criteria, as previously established [51].*
*ARVC may also be referred to as arrhythmogenic cardiomyopathy (ACM) [52].*

**Table 4.**
*Clinical findings and history are suggestive of a genetic evaluation.*

stratify cardiovascular risk, indicating the need for more aggressive lipid-lowering therapy. Positive genetic test results have also been shown to increase the initiation and adherence to lipid-lowering therapies, leading to reductions in LDLc [5].

### 2.1.1.4 Thoracic aortic aneurysm/dissection

Genetic testing has clinical utility for TAAD to inform syndromic disease management, such as a diagnosis of Marfan or Loeys-Dietz syndrome (which presents with TAAD). In addition, genetic testing informs aortic surgical decision-making by redefining thresholds for aortopathy management based on genetic testing results. Those with a TAAD molecular diagnosis may require earlier surgical intervention due to the increased risk of aortic events. For these patients, the surgical threshold for aortic root and ascending aortic aneurysms is often lower than the standard 5.5 cm, potentially reduced to 5.0 cm or even less [6].

**Table 1** of the AHA 2020 scientific statement provides the most comprehensive summary of the current knowledge on the clinical utility of genetic testing [1]; however, these claims are based on limited evidence and expert consensus rather than the evidence-based systematic approach recommended by the Institute of Medicine [53].

Evidence-based interventions are typically defined by their proven efficacy and effectiveness [54], with randomized controlled trials (RCTs) traditionally used to demonstrate efficacy [54]. However, no RCTs have been published to assess the efficacy of genetic testing. For example, there is a gap in the evidence supporting the effectiveness of genetic testing in the cardiomyopathy and arrhythmia literature. Non-guideline literature documenting the effectiveness, that is, whether genetic testing improves outcomes for patients, is also limited. The literature includes clinician-recommended actions such as device therapy, the initiation or intensification of medical therapies (e.g., oral anticoagulants or beta-blockers), advice on alcohol consumption and exercise, referrals to specialty clinics, initiation of drug treatments, and changes in care direction based on a metabolic or syndromic molecular diagnosis [55–63]. However, only two studies have reported on health outcomes related to these clinical actions. The first, by Rootwelt-Norberg et al. showed a reduction in ventricular arrhythmia after the implementation of genetic testing [61]. The second, by Ritter et al. (2020), reported an improvement in a syndromic cardiac condition following a riboflavin prescription [60].

### 2.1.2 Genetic counseling

Genetic counseling serves as a valuable resource in the genetic testing process, helping individuals get genetic testing and adapt to risk or a new diagnosis. Genetic counselors must be well-versed in guideline-directed recommendations to effectively communicate the benefits of genetic testing. Genetic counselors should also provide patients with education regarding genetic testing and the associated costs or insurance coverage details, the meaning of possible results, the limitations of genetic testing (e.g., detection rates are not 100%), and the family implications of genetic testing. They should also be prepared to provide psychological support and resources and to address concerns some patients express regarding confidentiality of results, such as having them in their medical records and available to insurance companies. A table is available (**Table 1**) in the article, *Evolving Cardiovascular Genetic Counseling Needs in the Era of Precision Medicine*, which summarizes key points to discuss when going through the informed consent process for CVD genetic testing [64]. In terms of communication strategies to address genetic testing and common patient concerns, patient-centric communication with active listening is key to understanding the patient's prior knowledge, context for any decisions or reactions, and comfort with the information the counselor is providing. Motivational interviewing or shared decision-making can be used to converse with patients about any decisions they have to make [65, 66]. Patients who present for genetic testing are dealing with their presenting symptoms and/or family history, and the fact that a genetic diagnosis could impact not only them but family also. They may have medical anxiety, and also financial anxiety related to the potential costs of testing and treatments. It is helpful to normalize and validate any feelings or concerns they share and offer support as needed and reassurance as appropriate. In the event that genetic testing yields a positive result, management recommendations should be reviewed in collaboration with the collaborating cardiologist to develop a care plan. **Table 5** illustrates the roles that genetic counselors play in addition to the management of cardiovascular genetic diseases [64].

### 2.1.3 Knowledge sharing between cardiologists and genetic counselors

Effective collaboration between genetic counselors and cardiologists is essential for identifying patients who require genetic testing and developing genetics-informed management plans. However, limited genetics education among cardiologists is a frequently cited barrier to cardiovascular genetic testing [67–72]. A survey of cardiology providers revealed that conducting risk assessments, implementing management strategies, ordering genetic tests, and interpreting results were highly desired topics for further education [73]. Genetic counselors are particularly competent in these areas, especially in conducting genetic risk assessments and managing genetic testing [74].

In addition to genetic counselors' complementary expertise to that of cardiologists, the Genetics Expertise and Analysis domain of the Practice Based Competencies

| Role | Description |
| --- | --- |
| Medical records review | Imaging, rhythm, history, and other clinical data are reviewed and discussed with the collaborating cardiologist to establish a cardiovascular genetic phenotype and rule out nongenetic etiologies (**Table 4**). |
| Pre- and post-test counseling | Explain testing processes, benefits and limitations, potential outcomes, and implications for medical management and family dynamics, offer psychosocial support, obtain informed consent, and interpret and communicate results. |
| Risk assessment and family screening | Obtain family history information using a targeted path of inquiry focused on heart disease, a patient-centered approach, and sensitivity to the potential psychological impact of discussing familial disease. Assess familial risk and guide cascade testing for at-risk relatives, select appropriate genetic tests interpret results in collaboration with the cardiologist, and recommend family testing in accordance with guidelines. |
| Emotional support and communication | Help patients cope with test results, and assist in communicating findings to family members. |
| Genetics-informed management | Review management recommendations in collaboration with the collaborating cardiologist to develop a care plan. |

**Table 5.**
*Genetic counselors' role in the management of cardiovascular genetic disease.*

of the Accreditation Council for Genetic Counseling includes principles of cardio-vascular genetics [75]. Still, there are limitations to this training because the depth of training can vary across programs. Therefore, genetic counselors primarily gain cardiology expertise through collaboration with cardiologists.

The Communities of Practice (CoP) model provides an excellent framework for collaboration between cardiologists and genetic counselors [76–78]. This model describes how groups learn together, generating tacit and explicit knowledge-sharing in cardiovascular genetics. Knowledge-sharing in a CoP context involves the exchange of information about genetics, cardiology, and approaches to clinical care of patients with heritable heart disease. This process integrates two disciplines, resulting in a broader understanding of patients. Knowledge-sharing can occur in various settings, including journal clubs, case conferences, and clinic conversations, among others.

Both genetic counselors and cardiologists benefit from knowledge-sharing by developing an enhanced view of their patients, potentially leading to improved patient experiences and health outcomes [79]. Role definition for the genetic counselor and the cardiologist in clinical practice settings is recommended. This recommendation is based on literature in other fields, which reported an association between role definition and positive team development. Trust is another key ingredient of effective teams. Team members should prioritize mutual interests, which may require giving up some autonomy [80]. In addition to role definition and trust, the Healthy Teams model identifies six indicators of health in clinical teams: mutual respect, goals, leadership, communication, cohesion, and purpose [81]. This model may be applied to the practice of cardiovascular genetics in the clinic.

## 2.2 Selecting the most appropriate test

Genetic testing in cardiovascular genetics encompasses various approaches, each with specific applications and considerations. The selection of the appropriate testing method depends on the clinical presentation, family history, and the specific cardiovascular condition under investigation. Current clinical testing modalities include:

1. Single gene testing: evaluates a specific gene known to be associated with a particular condition.

2. Panel testing: examines a group of genes associated with a specific cardiovascular condition or a set of related conditions.

3. Whole exome sequencing (WES): assesses almost all protein-coding sequences in the genome.

4. Whole genome sequencing (WGS): includes nearly all coding and noncoding sequences in the genome.

While cardiovascular genetics experts do not recommend a particular testing modality, they caution about the possibility of uninformative results when examining a large set of genes, particularly those with limited or refuted evidence [1]. In practice, most cardiovascular providers opt for panel testing [82, 83].

The choice of testing modality should be made in consultation with the collaborating cardiologist, taking into account the specific clinical context and the potential implications of the test results. When choosing a genetic test for cardiovascular disease, several factors should be considered [64]:

Panel testing

- Target specific gene variants associated with particular cardiovascular conditions (e.g., hypertrophic cardiomyopathy or arrhythmias)

- Ensure high informativeness

- Recommended for cases with clear clinical presentations

WES

- Useful when there's a strong suspicion of a genetic condition but the phenotype is unclear

- Appropriate when phenotype-specific panels do not provide a diagnosis

- Assesses almost all protein-coding sequences

WGS

- Offers comprehensive insights into both coding and noncoding sequences

- Considered when all other diagnostic tests are negative, but a strong suspicion of a genetic condition persists

- Provides the most extensive genetic information but may be more challenging to interpret

Despite multiple testing options, there are still patients who likely have underlying genetic causes for their symptoms that, despite testing, go undetected. This could be due to the fact that certain genomic regions are more poorly analyzed by standard genetic tests than other regions. Though not currently available for clinical use, third-generation "long read" sequencing has demonstrated potential in research settings and may be translated to clinical settings in the future [84].

## 2.3 Preparing patients for genetic testing (pre-test genetic counseling)

Due to the sensitive nature of genetic data, the limitations of the genetic tests available, the complexity of result interpretation, as well as the implications for other family members, it is important that patients are offered genetic counseling prior to cardiogenetic testing. Since cardiovascular genetic disease can be pediatric- or adult-onset, it is recommended that patients (and/or parents/guardians) receive pre-test counseling in an age-appropriate manner.

Key aspects of the process are discussed herein. As the healthcare provider prepares for the session, similar to all genetic counseling sessions, it is important to give special consideration to the selection of a private, quiet, comfortable environment that will help the patient feel safe and comfortable. A suitable environment can greatly facilitate the discussion of sensitive and potentially emotionally charged information. The discussion agenda needs to cover multiple topics, so as to both educate the patient as well as collect important information about them (**Table 6**). Toward

| Purpose | Discussion point | Content |
|---|---|---|
| Patient education | Explain the purpose of the session | E.g. facilitate a finite diagnosis, enable a prognosis, inform clinical management decisions, determine disease risk, guide reproductive choices. |
| | Ensure basic concepts are clarified | E.g. what DNA/genes, how they may contribute to disease presentation, and how they are inherited. |
| | Discuss suitable genetic testing options | E.g. what information they can provide, advantages and limitations, how they work, what the testing procedure involves (including the type of biological sample, collection procedure, basic aspects of DNA analysis methodology), time to results, how the results are communicated, lab options, cost, insurance coverage options. |
| | Present tentative impact of genetic testing results on other family members | E.g. depending on the findings other family members may be found to be at an increased risk of carrying the same pathogenic variant and/or at increased risk of presenting with the same disease. |
| | Address patient questions | E.g. scientific, technical, practical, concerns, fears. |
| Information collection | Collection of information on the family pedigree | Collect as detailed information as possible e.g. full list of at least three generations of blood relatives, members with a clinical diagnosis, undiagnosed members with symptoms, age at diagnosis/symptom presentation, deceased members with diagnosed or alleged symptoms -age and cause of death, any abortions (spontaneous or induced) and reasons. |
| | Assessment of patient familiarity with basic genetic testing concepts | E.g. the process of sample collection, what is analyzed, and what a genetic test can/cannot detect. |
| | Familiarity with the patient's cultural and religious beliefs | [Since these can influence their decision-making about testing and subsequent choices on course of action] |
| | Appreciation of the patient's current psychological status | E.g. fears, depression, traumas, prejudices, and misconception influencing their emotional response to the medical situation |

**Table 6.**
*General discussion points during the pre-test genetic counseling session.*

this direction gaining the patient's trust and building a line of open communication is key. The discussion agenda is best prepared ahead of time, but flexibility is recommended to enable adjustments to the individual's needs as they are unveiled during the genetic counseling session. Allowing the patient ample time to take in the new information and raise any concerns or questions they may have been valuable.

In cardiogenetic counseling, a number of additional, more specialized points need to be discussed.

The average detection rate of pathogenic/likely pathogenic variants is estimated to be approximately 40%. The identification of such a variant indicates disease causality and can be used for diagnostic/prognostic/management, as well as family cascade testing purposes.

The absence of a (likely) pathogenic variant in the gene panel tested, however, does not guarantee the absence of a pathogenic variant in other parts of the genome, and therefore cannot rule out the possibility of an inheritable form of CVD. In these instances, the use of an expanded gene panel or whole exome sequencing may be considered depending on the indications.

The identification of genetic variants of unknown significance is a frequent encounter, especially when larger cardio-gene panels or exome and whole genome sequencing are being used for testing [85]. Furthermore, in the case of the latter, large-scale testing approaches, the likelihood of incidental findings is significantly increased. These concepts are discussed in detail in the subsequent sections.

## 2.4 Access to genetic testing

Access to genetic testing and genetic services is not equal for all individuals and all geographic regions [86]. Many countries do not have enough genetic counselors or geneticists to meet population demand which can directly impact awareness of and availability of genetic testing. It can lead to long wait times and in some cases, patients seeking care from health professionals less skilled in discussing genetic testing and making genetic diagnoses. Additionally, very remote or rural areas may have less accessibility to healthcare facilities that offer genetic testing, necessitating long travel for those who are able. There may also be economic or policy barriers that impact access to genetic testing. Individuals in underserved communities may lack insurance or the financial means to pay out-of-pocket. In some regions, there may be policies or nationally funded healthcare that limit genetics testing options. In some communities, there are barriers to genetic testing because there are no educational resources available at all, or in the preferred language, to make community members aware of the benefits of genetic testing. Lastly, some individuals have cultural beliefs that affect their perception of the medical system, or they perceive a stigma around genetic diagnosis [87].

Genetic counselors can help to address disparities in access and care through education, outreach, augmented care models, and advocacy. Both at the personal and community level, they can endeavor to build trust. They can be a voice for patients and advocate for them by meeting with community leaders and organizations to establish or enhance connections and promote culturally sensitive and applicable availability of services. Many institutions and professional societies have recently focused on cultural competency within healthcare, and genetic counselors can take part in such training initiatives to empower them to understand and respect diverse backgrounds. There is a Genetic Counseling Cultural and Linguistic Competence Toolkit available online, created through funding awarded by the National Society of Genetic Counselors. There is an important role genetic counselors can play in increasing access to genetic testing by educating patients about their insurance coverage and potential requirements like prior authorization; they can make patients aware of financial assistance programs available through laboratories, healthcare institutions, or grants. They can also work to expand access to genetic counseling and genetic information by expanding and promoting telehealth options and other service delivery models, such as outreach clinics, e-consults, or genetic education modules in multiple languages. Last, efforts to reach and educate underserved populations can impact access to genetic services. Such efforts may include in-person or online information sessions, holding community workshops, or creating and disseminating materials tailored to specific cultural contexts. It is useful to consider community engagement in creating such material to ensure they are culturally relevant and appealing.

This section focused on incorporating genetic testing into routine clinical care and how genetic counselors are essential to this goal. Determining the need for genetic testing involves recognizing phenotypic traits associated with genetic causes of CVD. Effective collaboration between genetic counselors and cardiologists is important for identifying patients who require genetic testing and to guide effective clinical management. Genetic counseling is critical for preparing patients for testing, helping them understand potential results, and addressing emotional and ethical considerations. Barriers to genetic testing, such as access disparities and cultural factors must be addressed to ensure equitable testing availability.

## 3. Conclusions

In conclusion, the rapidly evolving field of CVD genetics holds tremendous promise for improving the prevention, diagnosis, and management of at-risk individuals and families. As genetic testing for CVD becomes more widespread, the role of specialized genetic counseling is increasingly critical in ensuring the appropriate use of testing, accurate interpretation of results, and meaningful integration of this information into clinical care. Pre-test genetic counseling is a crucial step in the effective implementation of cardiovascular genetic testing. It establishes a structured approach for assessing the appropriateness of testing, selecting the most relevant genetic assays, and ensuring patients and families are adequately informed about the potential outcomes and implications. This process enhances clinical decision-making, promotes patient autonomy, and lays the groundwork for integrating genetic insights into personalized care.

A close, interdisciplinary collaboration between cardiologists and genetic counselors is essential to create a cohesive framework that enhances decision-making and supports patients throughout the entire genetic testing process. Such collaboration ensures that complex genetic data is effectively translated into actionable clinical insights and that testing decisions are aligned with current guidelines and ethical considerations. As the field continues to advance, it will be essential to ensure that genetic counseling practices adapt to meet the growing demand for precision medicine approaches in cardiovascular healthcare.

## Acknowledgements

DS was supported by CUREPLaN, a grant from the Leducq Foundation for Cardiovascular Research (18CVD01).

## Conflict of interest

The authors declare no conflict of interest.

## Author details

Jessica Goehringer[1,2*], Despina Sanoudou[3*] and Ana Morales[1,4*]

1 Geisinger, Danville, PA, USA

2 Geisinger College of Health Sciences, Scranton, PA, USA

3 Clinical Genomics and Pharmacogenomics Unit, 4th Department of Internal Medicine, "Attikon" Hospital, Medical School, National and Kapodistrian University of Athens, Athens, Greece

4 The George Washington University, Translational Health Sciences Program, School of Medicine and Health Sciences, District of Columbia, USA

*Address all correspondence to: jgoehringer@geisinger.edu; dsanoudou@med.uoa.gr and amorales4@geisinger.edu

IntechOpen

# References

[1] Musunuru K, Hershberger RE, Day SM, Klinedinst NJ, Landstrom AP, Parikh VN, et al. Genetic testing for inherited cardiovascular diseases: A scientific statement from the American Heart Association. Circulation Genomic and Precision Medicine. 2020;**13**(4):e000067

[2] Wilde AAM, Semsarian C, Marquez MF, Shamloo AS, Ackerman MJ, Ashley EA, et al. European Heart Rhythm Association (EHRA)/Heart Rhythm Society (HRS)/ Asia Pacific Heart Rhythm Society (APHRS)/Latin American Heart Rhythm Society (LAHRS) Expert Consensus Statement on the state of genetic testing for cardiac diseases. Europace: European Pacing, Arrhythmias, and Cardiac Electrophysiology: Journal of the Working Groups on Cardiac Pacing, Arrhythmias, and Cardiac Cellular Electrophysiology of the European Society of Cardiology. 2022;**24**(8):1307-1367

[3] Hershberger RE, Givertz MM, Ho CY, Judge DP, Kantor PF, McBride KL, et al. Genetic evaluation of cardiomyopathy-a Heart Failure Society of America practice guideline. Journal of Cardiac Failure. 2018;**24**(5):281-302

[4] Brown EE, Sturm AC, Cuchel M, Braun LT, Duell PB, Underberg JA, et al. Genetic testing in dyslipidemia: A scientific statement from the National Lipid Association. Journal of Clinical Lipidology. 2020;**14**(4):398-413

[5] Sturm AC, Knowles JW, Gidding SS, Ahmad ZS, Ahmed CD, Ballantyne CM, et al. Clinical genetic testing for familial hypercholesterolemia: JACC scientific expert panel. Journal of the American College of Cardiology. 2018;**72**(6):662-680

[6] Writing Committee M, Isselbacher EM, Preventza O, Hamilton Black J III, Augoustides JG, Beck AW, et al. 2022 ACC/AHA guideline for the diagnosis and Management of Aortic Disease: A report of the American Heart Association/American College of Cardiology Joint Committee on Clinical Practice Guidelines. Journal of the American College of Cardiology. 2022;**80**(24):e223-e393

[7] Kassem H, Girolami F, Sanoudou D. Molecular genetics made simple. Global Cardiology Science & Practice. 2012;**2012**(1):6

[8] Srinivasan S, Won NY, Dotson WD, Wright ST, Roberts MC. Barriers and facilitators for cascade testing in genetic conditions: A systematic review. European Journal of Human Genetics: EJHG. 2020;**28**(12):1631-1644

[9] Gornick MC, Ryan KA, Scherer AM, Scott Roberts J, De Vries RG, Uhlmann WR. Interpretations of the term "actionable" when discussing genetic test results: What you mean is not what I heard. Journal of Genetic Counseling. 2019;**28**(2):334-342

[10] Richards S, Aziz N, Bale S, Bick D, Das S, Gastier-Foster J, et al. Standards and guidelines for the interpretation of sequence variants: A joint consensus recommendation of the American College of Medical Genetics and Genomics and the Association for Molecular Pathology. Genetics in Medicine: Official Journal of the American College of Medical Genetics. 2015;**17**(5):405-424

[11] Bowling KM, Thompson ML, Kelly MA, Scollon S, Slavotinek AM, Powell BC, et al. Return of non-ACMG

recommended incidental genetic findings to pediatric patients: Considerations and opportunities from experiences in genomic sequencing. Genome Medicine. 2022;**14**(1):131

[12] Schwartz MLB, McCormick CZ, Lazzeri AL, Lindbuchler DM, Hallquist MLG, Manickam K, et al. A model for genome-first Care: Returning secondary genomic findings to participants and their healthcare providers in a large research cohort. American Journal of Human Genetics. 2018;**103**(3):328-337

[13] Meng L, Attali R, Talmy T, Regev Y, Mizrahi N, Smirin-Yosef P, et al. Evaluation of an automated genome interpretation model for rare disease routinely used in a clinical genetic laboratory. Genetics in Medicine: Official Journal of the American College of Medical Genetics. 2023;**25**(6):100830

[14] Choi SW, Mak TS, O'Reilly PF. Tutorial: A guide to performing polygenic risk score analyses. Nature Protocols. 2020;**15**(9):2759-2772

[15] O'Sullivan JW, Raghavan S, Marquez-Luna C, Luzum JA, Damrauer SM, Ashley EA, et al. Polygenic risk scores for cardiovascular disease: A scientific statement from the American Heart Association. Circulation. 2022;**146**(8):e93-e118

[16] Phillips KA, Deverka PA, Hooker GW, Douglas MP. Genetic test availability and spending: Where are we now? Where are we going? Health Affairs. 2018;**37**(5):710-716

[17] Dorschner MO, Amendola LM, Turner EH, Robertson PD, Shirts BH, Gallego CJ, et al. Actionable, pathogenic incidental findings in 1,000 participants' exomes. American Journal of Human Genetics. 2013;**93**(4):631-640

[18] Foss KS, O'Daniel JM, Berg JS, Powell SN, Cadigan RJ, Kuczynski KJ, et al. The rise of population genomic screening: Characteristics of current programs and the need for evidence regarding optimal implementation. Journal of Personalized Medicine. 2022;**12**(5):1-17

[19] Archive C. Tier 1 Genomics Applications and their Importance to Public Health: CDC Archive; 2014. Available from: https://archive.cdc.gov/www_cdc_gov/genomics/implementation/toolkit/tier1.htm

[20] Guzauskas GF, Garbett S, Zhou Z, Schildcrout JS, Graves JA, Williams MS, et al. Population genomic screening for three common hereditary conditions : A cost-effectiveness analysis. Annals of Internal Medicine. 2023;**176**(5):585-595

[21] Jain CV, Kadam L, van Dijk M, Kohan-Ghadr HR, Kilburn BA, Hartman C, et al. Fetal genome profiling at 5 weeks of gestation after noninvasive isolation of trophoblast cells from the endocervical canal. Science Translational Medicine. 2016;**8**(363):363re4

[22] Pasquier L, Isidor B, Rial-Sebbag E, Odent S, Minguet G, Moutel G. Population genetic screening: Current issues in a European country. European Journal of Human Genetics: EJHG. 2019;**27**(9):1321-1323

[23] Stark Z, Schofield D, Martyn M, Rynehart L, Shrestha R, Alam K, et al. Does genomic sequencing early in the diagnostic trajectory make a difference? A follow-up study of clinical outcomes and cost-effectiveness. Genetics in Medicine: Official Journal of the American College of Medical Genetics. 2019;**21**(1):173-180

[24] Grzymski JJ, Elhanan G, Morales Rosado JA, Smith E, Schlauch KA,

Read F., et al. Population genetic screening efficiently identifies carriers of autosomal dominant diseases. Nature Medicine. 2020;**26**(8):1235-1239

[25] Abul-Husn NS, Soper ER, Braganza GT, Rodriguez JE, Zeid N, Cullina S, et al. Implementing genomic screening in diverse populations. Genome Medicine. 2021;**13**(1):17

[26] Carey DJ, Fetterolf SN, Davis FD, Faucett WA, Kirchner HL, Mirshahi U, et al. The Geisinger MyCode community health initiative: An electronic health record-linked biobank for precision medicine research. Genetics in Medicine: Official Journal of the American College of Medical Genetics. 2016;**18**(9):906-913

[27] David SP, Dunnenberger HM, Ali R, Matsil A, Lemke AA, Singh L, et al. Implementing primary care mediated population genetic screening within an integrated health system. Journal of the American Board of Family Medicine: JABFM. 2021;**34**(4):861-865

[28] Williams MS. Population screening in health systems. Annual Review of Genomics and Human Genetics. 2022;**23**:549-567

[29] Kelly MA, Leader JB, Wain KE, Bodian D, Oetjens MT, Ledbetter DH, et al. Leveraging population-based exome screening to impact clinical care: The evolution of variant assessment in the Geisinger MyCode research project. American Journal of Medical Genetics Part C, Seminars in Medical Genetics. 2021;**187**(1):83-94

[30] Miller DT, Lee K, Abul-Husn NS, Amendola LM, Brothers K, Chung WK, et al. ACMG SF v3.2 list for reporting of secondary findings in clinical exome and genome sequencing: A policy statement of the American College of Medical Genetics and Genomics (ACMG).

Genetics in Medicine : Official Journal of the American College of Medical Genetics. 2023;**25**(8):100866

[31] Buchanan AH, Lester Kirchner H, Schwartz MLB, Kelly MA, Schmidlen T, Jones LK, et al. Clinical outcomes of a genomic screening program for actionable genetic conditions. Genetics in Medicine: Official Journal of the American College of Medical Genetics. 2020;**22**(11):1874-1882

[32] Collaboration EASFHS, Vallejo-Vaz AJ, De Marco M, Stevens CAT, Akram A, Freiberger T, et al. Overview of the current status of familial hypercholesterolaemia care in over 60 countries - The EAS Familial Hypercholesterolaemia Studies Collaboration (FHSC). Atherosclerosis. 2018;**277**:234-255

[33] Nordestgaard BG, Chapman MJ, Humphries SE, Ginsberg HN, Masana L, Descamps OS, et al. Familial hypercholesterolaemia is underdiagnosed and undertreated in the general population: Guidance for clinicians to prevent coronary heart disease: Consensus statement of the European Atherosclerosis Society. European Heart Journal. 2013;**34**(45):3478-390a

[34] Representatives of the Global Familial Hypercholesterolemia C, Wilemon KA, Patel J, Aguilar-Salinas C, Ahmed CD, Alkhnifsawi M, et al. Reducing the clinical and public health burden of familial hypercholesterolemia: A global call to action. JAMA Cardiology. 2020;**5**(2):217-229

[35] Rao ND, Kaganovsky J, Malouf EA, Coe S, Huey J, Tsinajinne D, et al. Diagnostic yield of genetic screening in a diverse, community-ascertained cohort. Genome Medicine. 2023;**15**(1):26

[36] Joly Y, Dalpe G. Genetic discrimination still casts a large shadow

in 2022. European Journal of Human Genetics: EJHG. 2022;**30**(12):1320-1322

[37] Joly Y, Dupras C, Pinkesz M, Tovino SA, Rothstein MA. Looking beyond GINA: Policy approaches to address genetic discrimination. Annual Review of Genomics and Human Genetics. 2020;**21**:491-507

[38] Hershberger RE, Jordan E. Dilated Cardiomyopathy Overview. University of Washington, Seattle: GeneReviews(®); 1993

[39] Vasan RS, Larson MG, Levy D, Evans JC, Benjamin EJ. Distribution and categorization of echocardiographic measurements in relation to reference limits: The Framingham Heart Study: Formulation of a height- and sex-specific classification and its prospective validation. Circulation. 1997;**96**(6):1863-1873

[40] Cirino AL, Ho C. Hypertrophic Cardiomyopathy Overview. University of Washington, Seattle: GeneReviews(®); 1993

[41] McNally E, MacLeod H, Dellefave-Castillo L. Arrhythmogenic Right Ventricular Cardiomyopathy Overview. University of Washington, Seattle: GeneReviews(®); 1993

[42] Kamath GS, Zareba W, Delaney J, Koneru JN, McKenna W, Gear K, et al. Value of the signal-averaged electrocardiogram in arrhythmogenic right ventricular cardiomyopathy/dysplasia. Heart Rhythm. 2011;**8**(2):256-262

[43] Cimiotti D, Budde H, Hassoun R, Jaquet K. Genetic restrictive cardiomyopathy: Causes and consequences-an integrative approach. International Journal of Molecular Sciences. 2021;**22**(2):1-26

[44] Muchtar E, Blauwet LA, Gertz MA. Restrictive cardiomyopathy: Genetics, pathogenesis, clinical manifestations, diagnosis, and therapy. Circulation Research. 2017;**121**(7):819-837

[45] Groffen AJ, Bikker H, Christiaans I. Long QT Syndrome Overview. University of Washington, Seattle: GeneReviews(®); 1993

[46] Napolitano C, Mazzanti A, Bloise R, Priori SG. Catecholaminergic Polymorphic Ventricular Tachycardia. University of Washington, Seattle: GeneReviews(®); 1993

[47] Brugada R, Campuzano O, Sarquella-Brugada G, et al. Brugada Syndrome. In: Adam MP, Feldman J, Mirzaa GM, et al., editors. GeneReviews® [Internet]. Seattle (WA): University of Washington, Seattle; 2005 Mar 31 [Updated 2022 Aug 25]. 1993-2024. Available from: https://nam12.safelinks.protection.outlook.com/?url=https%3A%2F%2Fwww.ncbi.nlm.nih.gov%2Fbooks%2FNBK1517%2F&data=05%7C02%7Cjgoehringer%40geisinger.edu%7Cbabfe46bdd61439a675808dd0b333103%7C37d46c567c664402a16055c2313b910d%7C0%7C0%7C638679036666903457%7CUnknown%7CTWFpbGZsb3d8eyJFbXB0eU1hcGkiOnRydWUsIlYiOiIwLjAwMDAiLCJAiO iJXaW4zMiIsIkFOIjoiTWFpbCIsIldUIjoyfQ%3D%3D%7C0%7C%7C%7C&sdata=29GZalWaj%2Fuvcs DrauUUOZ%2BCz3a21fDu3zOHP6bSrSI%3D&reserved=0

[48] Milewicz DM, Cecchi AC. Heritable THORACIc Aortic Disease Overview. University of Washington, Seattle: GeneReviews(®); 1993

[49] Campens L, Demulier L, De Groote K, Vandekerckhove K, De Wolf D,

Romar MJ, et al. Reference values for echocardiographic assessment of the diameter of the aortic root and ascending aorta spanning all age categories. The American Journal of Cardiology. 2014;**114**(6):914-920

[50] Devereux RB, de Simone G, Arnett DK, Best LG, Boerwinkle E, Howard BV, et al. Normal limits in relation to age, body size and gender of two-dimensional echocardiographic aortic root dimensions in persons >/=15 years of age. The American Journal of Cardiology. 2012;**110**(8):1189-1194

[51] Marcus FI, McKenna WJ, Sherrill D, Basso C, Bauce B, Bluemke DA, et al. Diagnosis of arrhythmogenic right ventricular cardiomyopathy/dysplasia: Proposed modification of the task force criteria. European Heart Journal. 2010;**31**(7):806-814

[52] Towbin JA, McKenna WJ, Abrams DJ, Ackerman MJ, Calkins H, Darrieux FCC, et al. 2019 HRS expert consensus statement on evaluation, risk stratification, and management of arrhythmogenic cardiomyopathy. Heart Rhythm. 2019;**16**(11):e301-ee72

[53] Institute of Medicine · Board on Health Care Services, Guidelines CoSfDTCP. Clinical Practice Guidelines We Can Trust. Washington, DC: National Academis Press; 2011

[54] Grol R, Wensing M, Eccles M, Davis D. Implementation of Change in Healthcare: A Complex Problem. Improving Patient Care: The Implementation of Change in Health Care. 2nd ed. Oxford, UK: Wiley-Blackwell; 2013

[55] Amin RJ, Morris-Rosendahl D, Edwards M, Tayal U, Buchan R, Hammersley DJ, et al. The addition of genetic testing and cardiovascular

magnetic resonance to routine clinical data for stratification of etiology in dilated cardiomyopathy. Frontiers in Cardiovascular Medicine. 2022;**9**:1017119

[56] Broch K, Andreassen AK, Hopp E, Leren TP, Scott H, Muller F, et al. Results of comprehensive diagnostic work-up in 'idiopathic' dilated cardiomyopathy. Open Heart. 2015;**2**(1):e000271

[57] Hoss S, Habib M, Silver J, Care M, Chan RH, Hanneman K, et al. Genetic testing for diagnosis of hypertrophic cardiomyopathy mimics: Yield and clinical significance. Circulation Genomic and Precision Medicine. 2020;**13**(2):e002748

[58] Maestro-Benedicto A, Vela P, de Frutos F, Mora N, Pomares A, Gonzalez-Vioque E, et al. Frequency of hereditary transthyretin amyloidosis among elderly patients with transthyretin cardiomyopathy. European Journal of Heart Failure. 2022;**24**(12):2367-2373

[59] Neves R, Bains S, Bos JM, MacIntyre C, Giudicessi JR, Ackerman MJ. Precision therapy in congenital long QT syndrome. Trends in Cardiovascular Medicine. 2024;**34**(1):39-47

[60] Ritter A, Bedoukian E, Berger JH, Copenheaver D, Gray C, Krantz I, et al. Clinical utility of exome sequencing in infantile heart failure. Genetics in Medicine: Official Journal of the American College of Medical Genetics. 2020;**22**(2):423-426

[61] Rootwelt-Norberg C, Lie OH, Dejgaard LA, Chivulescu M, Leren IS, Edvardsen T, et al. Life-threatening arrhythmic presentation in patients with arrhythmogenic cardiomyopathy before and after entering the genomic era; a two-decade experience from a large

volume center. International Journal of Cardiology. 2019;**279**:79-83

[62] Rosenzweig A, Watkins H, Hwang DS, Miri M, McKenna W, Traill TA, et al. Preclinical diagnosis of familial hypertrophic cardiomyopathy by genetic analysis of blood lymphocytes. The New England Journal of Medicine. 1991;**325**(25):1753-1760

[63] Smith E, Thompson PD, Burke-Martindale C, Weissler-Snir A. Establishment of a dedicated inherited cardiomyopathy clinic: From challenges to improved patients' outcome. Journal of the American Heart Association. 2022;**11**(9):e024501

[64] Morales A, Goehringer J, Sanoudou D. Evolving cardiovascular genetic counseling needs in the era of precision medicine. Frontiers in Cardiovascular Medicine. 2023;**10**:1161029

[65] Birch PH, Adam S, Coe RR, Port AV, Vortel M, Friedman JM, et al. Assessing shared decision-making clinical behaviors among genetic counsellors. Journal of Genetic Counseling. Feb 2019;**28**(1):40-49

[66] Spector A, Ash E, Garland B, McLaughlin R, Ritenour A, Gonynor C, et al. Perceptions of motivational interviewing in genetic counseling practice and training. Journal of Genetic Counseling. 2022;**31**(5):1173-1182

[67] Arrobas Velilla T, Brea A, Valdivielso P. Implementation of a biochemical, clinical, and genetic screening programme for familial hypercholesterolemia in 26 centres in Spain: The ARIAN study. Frontiers in Genetics. 2022;**13**:971651

[68] Bonter K, Desjardins C, Currier N, Pun J, Ashbury FD. Personalised

medicine in Canada: A survey of adoption and practice in oncology, cardiology and family medicine. BMJ Open. 2011;**1**(1):e000110

[69] Christensen KD, Vassy JL, Jamal L, Lehmann LS, Slashinski MJ, Perry DL, et al. Are physicians prepared for whole genome sequencing? A qualitative analysis. Clinical Genetics. 2016;**89**(2):228-234

[70] Hamilton AB, Oishi S, Yano EM, Gammage CE, Marshall NJ, Scheuner MT. Factors influencing organizational adoption and implementation of clinical genetic services. Genetics in Medicine: Official Journal of the American College of Medical Genetics. 2014;**16**(3):238-245

[71] Miller DM, Gaviglio A, Zierhut HA. Development of an implementation framework for overcoming underdiagnoses of familial hypercholesterolemia in the USA. Public Health Genomics. 2021;**24**(3-4):110-122

[72] Will CM, Armstrong D, Marteau TM. Genetic unexceptionalism: Clinician accounts of genetic testing for familial hypercholesterolaemia. Social Science & Medicine. 2010;**71**(5):910-917

[73] Lopez Santibanez Jacome L, Dellefave-Castillo LM, Wicklund CA, Scherr CL, Duquette D, Webster G, et al. Practitioners' confidence and desires for education in cardiovascular and sudden cardiac death genetics. Journal of the American Heart Association. 2022;**11**(7):e023763

[74] Arscott P, Caleshu C, Kotzer K, Kreykes S, Kruisselbrink T, Orland K, et al. A case for inclusion of genetic counselors in cardiac care. Cardiology in Review. 2016;**24**(2):49-55

[75] Counseling AACfGCACfG. ACGC Practice Based Competencies - Forms &

Resources. 2022. Available from: https://www.gceducation.org/forms-resources/

[76] Cantillon P, D'Eath M, De Grave W, Dornan T. How do clinicians become teachers? A communities of practice perspective. Advances in Health Sciences Education: Theory and Practice. 2016;**21**(5):991-1008

[77] Ranmuthugala G, Plumb JJ, Cunningham FC, Georgiou A, Westbrook JI, Braithwaite J. How and why are communities of practice established in the healthcare sector? A systematic review of the literature. BMC Health Services Research. 2011;**11**:273

[78] Wenger E. Communities of practice and social learning systems: The career of a concept. In: Blackmore C, editor. Social Learning Systems and Communities of Practice. London, UK: Springer; 2010. pp. 179-198

[79] Oben P. Understanding the patient experience: A conceptual framework. Journal of Patient Experience. 2020;**7**(6):906-910

[80] Bennett LM, Gadlin H. Collaboration and team science: From theory to practice. Journal of Investigative Medicine: The Official Publication of the American Federation for Clinical Research. 2012;**60**(5):768-775

[81] Mickan SM, Rodger SA. Effective health care teams: A model of six characteristics developed from shared perceptions. Journal of Interprofessional Care. 2005;**19**(4):358-370

[82] Kalayinia S, Goodarzynejad H, Maleki M, Mahdieh N. Next generation sequencing applications for cardiovascular disease. Annals of Medicine. 2018;**50**(2):91-109

[83] Lebo MS, Baxter SM. New molecular genetic tests in the diagnosis of heart disease. Clinics in Laboratory Medicine. 2014;**34**(1):137-156, vii-viii

[84] Olivucci G, Iovino E, Innella G, Turchetti D, Pippucci T, Magini P. Long read sequencing on its way to the routine diagnostics of genetic diseases. Frontiers in Genetics. 2024;**15**:1374860

[85] Chen E, Facio FM, Aradhya KW, Rojahn S, Hatchell KE, Aguilar S, et al. Rates and classification of variants of uncertain significance in hereditary disease genetic testing. JAMA Network Open. 2023;**6**(10):e2339571

[86] Williams JK, Bonham VL, Wicklund C, Coleman B, Taylor JY, Cashion AK. Advocacy and actions to address disparities in access to genomic health care: A report on a National Academies workshop. Nursing Outlook. 2019;**67**(5):605-612

[87] Baynam G, Gomez R, Jain R. Stigma associated with genetic testing for rare diseases-causes and recommendations. Frontiers in Genetics. 2024;**15**:1335768

Chapter 3

# Genetic Counseling for Cardiovascular Disease: Part B – Post-Test Approaches and Considerations

*Despina Sanoudou, Jessica Goehringer and Ana Morales*

## Abstract

With the increasing availability and adoption of genetic testing in cardiovascular disease (CVD), effective post-testing management is becoming crucial for optimizing patient outcomes and providing personalized care. This chapter focuses on key strategies and considerations for interpreting genetic test results in CVD, navigating complex scenarios such as incidental findings (IFs) and variants of unknown significance (VUS), and utilizing advanced tools and databases for evidence-based interpretation. As genetic testing becomes more integrated into routine clinical practice, the ability to communicate results clearly and accurately to patients and their families is paramount. This chapter provides practical guidance on delivering genetic information in a clinically meaningful way while adhering to international recommendations and addressing sensitive issues like non-paternity disclosure and risk assessment for family members through cascade testing. Special attention is given to the unique challenges of testing minors and the ethical frameworks that guide these decisions. Finally, the chapter addresses the psychosocial implications of CVD genetic testing and offers support strategies to help patients and families navigate the impact of their results. As the field of CVD genetics continues to expand, this comprehensive approach is essential for translating genetic data into actionable insights that enhance patient care and family health management.

**Keywords:** cardiovascular disease, genetic disease, genetic counseling, genetic testing, cardiovascular genetics, cardiogenetics, cardiogenomics, laboratory genetics, personalized medicine, precision medicine, gene panels, next generation sequencing, cardiomyopathies, arrhythmias, familial hypercholesterolemia, thoracic aortic aneurysm, dissection

## 1. Introduction

Genetic counseling for cardiovascular disease (CVD) extends beyond the decision to pursue testing and encompasses a critical post-testing phase, where complex genetic information must be accurately interpreted and communicated. This chapter focuses on the key considerations and strategies for managing genetic test results in clinical practice. Central to this process is the correct interpretation of genetic testing results, the use of specialized tools and databases, and the management of findings such as incidental results and variants of unknown significance (VUS). While variant classification is performed by the genetic testing laboratory, each of these elements requires a comprehensive understanding of genetics and meticulous attention to detail by the clinician, as misinterpretation of a result can lead to misguided clinical decisions.

Equally important is the effective communication of genetic results to patients and their families. Conveying the implications of genetic findings involves not only explaining the technical aspects but also addressing sensitive issues like non-paternity or risk determination for family members through cascade testing. This chapter further examines special considerations when dealing with minors and highlights the ethical frameworks that guide these discussions. Ultimately, post-testing genetic counseling is about bridging the gap between complex genomic data and patient care, ensuring that the results are integrated meaningfully into health management strategies while supporting families through the emotional and ethical challenges that may arise.

## 2. Key aspects of post-testing CVD genetic counseling

A multitude of specialized genetic tests have been developed to detect pathogenic variants implicated in cardiovascular diseases (CVDs). These tests typically involve sequencing of targeted gene panels, which can range from a single gene to more than three hundred genes, and in certain diagnostically challenging cases, may extend to whole exome sequencing (WES) to uncover the underlying genetic etiology. The selection of the appropriate genetic test is determined by the clinical context: a focused panel may be used when a specific pathogenic variant is suspected, while a broader gene panel or WES may be employed in cases with complex or ambiguous phenotypes where multiple genes or pathways could be involved. In the authors' experience, the CVD conditions for which genetic testing referrals are more frequently made include cardiomyopathies, arrhythmias, familial hypercholesterolemia, and aortopathies. The results derived from cardiogenetic testing provide critical insights for establishing a definitive diagnosis, refining risk stratification, and guiding individualized clinical management. Furthermore, these findings enable the identification of additional at-risk relatives through cascade testing, thereby facilitating timely surveillance and preventive strategies within affected families. However, the interpretation, communication, and follow-up of the findings require relevant expertise and careful consideration. Key aspects of the post-testing CVD genetic counseling process are discussed in detail in the subsequent sections.

### 2.1 Variant interpretation

When interpreting, discussing, or delivering the results of genetic testing in a clinical or research environment, one must understand the preferred terminology. Historically, the terms used to describe variation from the reference DNA sequence were "mutation" (i.e., a permanent change in the nucleotide sequence) and "polymorphism" (i.e., a common variant in a specific sequence of DNA, where "common" is typically defined as an allele frequency of at least 1% in the general population) [1].

These terms have now largely been retired since not every mutation confers a negative or disease-causing change and not every polymorphism is benign.

Instead, several professional organizations recommend using the term "variant" to describe a change from the reference DNA sequence. Modifiers are then added to clearly define how the variant is predicted to impact the function of a gene and, therefore, the phenotype. These modifiers are part of a widely used variant classification system introduced in 2015 when stakeholders from the American College of Medical Genetics and Genomics (ACMG), the Association for Molecular Pathology (AMP), and the College of American Pathologists (CAP) released guidelines for the interpretation of sequence variants [1].

### 2.1.1 Sequence variants

The guidelines recommend using the following terms as modifiers to define sequence variants identified in Mendelian disorders via single gene testing, panel testing, whole exome, or whole genome sequencing:

Pathogenic (P): Enough evidence to indicate, with certainty, a variant is causing a disease.

Likely pathogenic (LP): Greater than 90% certainty of a variant being disease-causing.

Likely benign (LB): Greater than 90% certainty of a variant being benign.

Benign (B): Enough evidence to indicate, with certainty, a variant is not causing a disease.

Uncertain significance (VUS): Not enough evidence to be classified as P/LP or LB/B.

Variant classification into these five categories is based on identifying the variant and gathering information (e.g., population data, functional data, segregation data, computational data, disease databases, and medical and scientific literature) that gets assimilated into a final classification decision. The 2015 "Standards and Guidelines for the Interpretation of Sequence Variants" review twenty-eight different evidence types and assigns each a weight [1]. The evidence types are divided into two categories: (1) those that contribute to a pathogenic interpretation or (2) those that contribute to a benign interpretation. Weighting of the evidence types within each category ranges from strong to supporting for benign interpretations to supporting, moderate, strong, or very strong for pathogenic interpretations. There is a very useful chart that organizes criteria by strength and type of evidence available at [2].

In addition to the guidelines for classifying sequence variants in Mendelian genes, there are guidelines available for variant interpretation of mitochondrial DNA (mtDNA) and copy number variants (CNVs) that consider the unique factors inherent to both [2, 3].

Diseases caused by variants in the mtDNA, including those that can contribute to mitochondrial cardiomyopathy and heart failure, are both phenotypically and genetically heterogeneous, posing challenges for diagnosis and management [4]. Factors impacting variant interpretation of the mitochondrial genome include maternal inheritance, variant heteroplasmy (having more than one mitochondrial genome per cell, with fluctuations in the number of genomes in a given tissue over time), the threshold effect (the proportion of wild-type mtDNA to mtDNA with a variant), and other complexities. The "Specifications of the ACMG/AMP Standards and Guidelines for Mitochondrial DNA Variant Interpretation" uses the same five-tier classification system (P/LP/VUS/LB/B) as the ACMG/AMP 2015 Guidelines for sequence variants.

However, relevance to mtDNA for all rules resulted in nineteen rules with further specifications related to mtDNA, and seven rules were removed due to their lack of applicability to mtDNA. For a detailed summary of the updated evidence rules, please refer to the guidelines.

### 2.1.2 Copy number variants

Copy number variants (CNVs) are genomic gains (duplications or multiplications) and losses (deletions), which can be associated with physiological human variation or pathological phenotypes. CNVs have been implicated in cases of cardiomyopathies and arrhythmia syndromes, as well as familial hypercholesterolemia, aortopathy, and sudden cardiac death [5, 6] (DOI: 10.1194/jlr.D079301; DOI: 10.1038/gim.2015.88).

Most CNVs are unique, requiring careful assessment to determine whether they are clinically significant. In 2020, in collaboration with the National Institutes of Health (NIH)-funded Clinical Genome Resource (ClinGen) project, the ACMG developed professional standards to support clinical laboratories in classifying and reporting CNVs [3]. Evidence categories pertaining to CNV classifications were decided (e.g., genomic content, dosage sensitivity predictions and curations, predicted functional effect, clinical overlap with patients in the medical literature, evidence from case and control databases, and inheritance patterns for individual CNVs). The guidelines call for assigning a relative weight to each evidence category to form a semiquantitative point-based scoring system with five tiers. Scores for each category of evidence are summed. Those in support of pathogenicity are positive values, and those refuting pathogenicity are negative values. The final classification, based on point values, is as follows:

$\geq 0.99$ point value: Pathogenic, strong evidence of pathogenicity.

0.90 to 0.98 point value: Likely pathogenic, strong evidence suggests CNV will ultimately be classified as disease-causing

$-0.89$ to 0.89 point value: VUS, at time of reporting, there was insufficient evidence to determine the clinical significance of the CNV.

$-0.90$ to $-0.98$ point value: Likely benign, strong evidence to suggest CNV is not involved in Mendelian disease.

$\leq -0.99$ point value: Benign, strong evidence from peer-reviewed publications or databases as non-disease-causing; may represent a benign polymorphism.

For a detailed summary of the evidence categories, how to apply them, and special considerations, please refer to the Guidelines [3].

### 2.1.3 Variant classification and reclassification

As the goal with genetic testing is identifying the cause of signs and symptoms comprising a phenotype in an individual, an accurate variant classification has major implications for clinical care. The standardization of variant interpretation is intended to provide transparency and consistency across laboratories, thereby reducing the frequency of differing variant classification and increasing the accuracy of genetic diagnoses. However, it is possible for different laboratories to view the same variant in a gene yet classify the variant differently, likely because of looking at different evidence or applying different weights to levels of evidence criteria. If a clinician (including physicians, advanced practitioners, genetic counselors, etc.) questions the variant classification for a given patient based on cardiac clinical and family history, performing their own research through literature or database review (see next section) on the identified variant is prudent, as is contacting the lab to discuss the classification approach used. Sometimes this can lead to a change in the variant classification and genetic test report, with tentatively significant clinical implications.

The expanding use of genomic sequencing leads to the detection of an increasing number of rare or novel DNA variants, often classified as VUS. This can be challenging because it may leave the clinician and the patient with an unclear answer regarding diagnosis and CVD management. Although a variety of tools are available to evaluate the overall weight of benign and pathogenic evidence of a VUS, it's important to note that a VUS classification should not be used by clinicians to make clinical decisions about the patient or at-risk relatives [1]. Instead, it's recommended that clinical investigation, such as family studies, and accumulating evidence to aid in reclassification of the variant be pursued to determine the level of pathogenicity of a variant.

As scientific knowledge evolves, sequencing upon genome reanalysis improves, and bioinformatics pipelines are updated, genetic variants can be reclassified. This is especially the case for VUS, but it can occur within and between any category of classification (P/LP/VUS/LB/B). Because genomic knowledge rapidly advances, for some types of testing, such as WES, certain laboratories offer a reanalysis of the sequence data, best performed at minimum 2 years after initial variant classification. Current literature shows that variant reclassification rates range from 3.6 to 58.8% depending on conditions and causes [7–9]. Of note, there are varying opinions on whether the laboratory or ordering clinician are responsible for re-investigating and updating variant status.

### 2.1.4 Tools and databases

There are a variety of tools and databases publicly and freely available to aid in the interpretation of genomic variants, while others are pay-for-use models. Different genetics laboratories may use one or more of these tools to assist with variant classification and/or may develop their own classification algorithms and databases. Reference population databases to assist in variant interpretation as population frequency data enable users to separate rare variants more likely to be the cause of Mendelian disease from common, generally benign variants [10]. The list provided in **Table 1** represents a selection of some of the more widely used and freely available resources.

Of note, genomic data have historically been aggregated largely from individuals of European descent, which is a barrier when conducting variant interpretation from underrepresented populations. Though population databases are making considerable progress in including diverse datasets, there are substantial gaps for individuals who are not of White European race/ethnic/ancestry groups, leading to higher VUS rates in non-White European groups [7].

## 2.2 Incidental and secondary findings

Beyond the genetic findings that are directly related to the disease tested for, incidental or secondary findings of medical value (actionable findings) for patient care may be discovered (**Table 1**). Although the terms incidental findings (IF) and secondary findings (SF) have long (and still to a certain extent) been used interchangeably, a distinction between the two has now been introduced. The terms incidental or unsolicited findings refer to genetic findings that have medical relevance but are not related to the indication for testing and not intentionally sought during analysis [11]. Secondary findings are also unrelated to the indication for testing, but they are identified as a result of a deliberate search for medically relevant variants [12].

| Resource | Description | Available at |
|---|---|---|
| **Interpretation calculators** | | |
| ClinGen pathogenicity calculator for variant classification | Using the 2015 ACMG/AMP Standards and Guidelines for the Interpretation of Sequence Variants, this calculator allows for the automatic calculation of a provisional conclusion based on the most current evidence. It provides applicable rules, evidence codes, and links to supporting data to detail the reasoning behind the conclusion. The calculator can generate a report printable as a PDF and provide URL links for sharing. | Pathogenicity Calculator (clinicalgenome.org) |
| ClinGen CNV interpretation calculator | This tool is based on the CNV scoring metrics that appear in the 2020 ACMG Technical Standards for the Interpretation and Reporting of Constitutional Copy Number Variants. It is designed to help the user track and sum the points they assigned to each level of criteria to arrive at a preliminary CNV classification. CNV Scoring Rubrics are available for copy number loss and gains. | CNV Pathogenicity Calculator (clinicalgenome.org) Loss: CNV Pathogenicity Calculator (clinicalgenome.org) Gains: CNV Pathogenicity Calculator (clinicalgenome.org) |
| CNV-ClinViewer | This is a web application offered through the Broad Institute in Boston, Massachusetts, USA, that allows for semi-automated clinical significance classification of CNVs based on the 2019 ACMG/ClinGen Technical Standards for CNVs. It generates CNV reports that note the clinical significance classification and associated annotation details. | https://cnv-clinviewer. broadinstitute.org |
| **Reference population databases** | | |
| Genome Aggregation Database (gnomAD) | This is the largest and most widely accessed reference population dataset, developed by an international coalition of investigators to aggregate and harmonize exome and genome sequencing data. It is searchable by gene, region, or variant. | gnomAD (broadinstitute.org) |
| Trans-Omics for Precision Medicine (TOPMed) | The TOPMed Program collects genomic, proteomic, and metabolomic data and integrates it with molecular, behavioral, imaging, environmental, and clinical data to advance efforts in the prevention and treatment of heart, lung, blood, and sleep disorders. The database contains clinical data and whole genome sequences of those with European ancestry (about 40%) and non-European ancestry (about 60%). There are open-access datasets (e.g., 1000 Genomes Project) available through the NHLBI BioData Catalyst (BDC). | Join the BDC Community \| BDC (nih.gov) |
| **Other tools, databases, repositories, and archives** | | |
| DECIPHER | This is a web-based database intended for the deposition, analysis, and sharing of potentially pathogenic variants from patients with rare genetic disorders who have been carefully phenotyped. It has an international community of academic and clinical genetic contributors, culminating in thousands of submitted cases. DECIPHER provides tools to users to assist with variant analysis and identification of other patients showing similar genotype–phenotype characteristics. | DECIPHER v11.26: Mapping the clinical genome (deciphergenomics.org) |

| Resource | Description | Available at |
|---|---|---|
| ClinGen Evidence Repository | This is a United States Food and Drug Administration (FDA)-recognized human genetic variant database that contains expert-curated assertions regarding a variant's pathogenicity and includes supporting evidence summaries. It is searchable by gene, disease, and variant. | Evidence Repository - Clinical Genome Resources |
| ClinVar | Maintained by the United States National Institutes of Health (NIH), ClinVar is a partner of the ClinGen project and a public archive of human genetic variants and interpretations of how they are related to disease. Anyone can submit an interpretation of a variant, ideally with supporting evidence describing the criteria they use to classify variants. Users can search submitted data and summary data for a given genetic disease or variant. | ClinVar (nih.gov) |
| GeniE | The Genetic Prevalence Estimator, supported by the Broad Institute and Chan Zuckerberg Initiative, uses data from open-source databases (e.g., ClinVar and gnomAD) to help users estimate the prevalence for recessive diseases. | About Genetic Prevalence Estimator (broadinstitute.org) |

**Table 1.**
*Free and publicly available tools and databases used in the interpretation of genomic variants.*

The frequency of IF/SF is rapidly increasing along with the expanding use of large-scale sequencing. These findings can have a significant impact on patients' and their family lives, ranging from unnecessary anxiety to pre-symptomatic disease detection and prevention. However, determining if, when, and how these findings should be communicated to the patient is highly challenging (see Section 2.3 Communication of genetic test results).

Although with targeted variant and disease-specific gene panel testing it is unlikely to observe IFs, in other cases, such as when exome or whole genome sequencing is ordered, the frequency of IFs can be significantly higher. For example, meta-analysis of whole genome sequencing (WGS) and WES data estimates a frequency of actionable IFs of 0.59–10.3% across the fifty-nine gene lists recommended at the time by ACMG for reporting [13]. Similarly, a subsequent study of 21,915 individuals estimated an IFs' frequency of 2.54% for the same fifty-nine ACMG genes [14].

It should be noted that the detection of IFs can be significantly different across populations. For example, in one meta-analysis, the frequency was 50% lower in African populations, likely due to the poor representation of the African genome in the international databases [13]. This calls for increased caution during the interpretation of variant findings across different population groups.

Beyond the ACMG recommendations on the return of these findings (see Section 2.3 Communication of genetic test results), challenges remain regarding the identification, interpretation, and return of IFs to patients. This process can be further complicated by parameters such as variable expressivity, reduced penetrance, or the discovery of novel variants. Initiatives such as the Electronic Medical Records and Genomics (eMERGE) network and the Clinical Sequencing Exploratory Research (CSER) consortium are working toward the integration of genetic information into electronic medical records. This could facilitate healthcare provider access to the patients' genetic results, but at the same time it will increase the frequency and complexity of the genetic information requiring interpretation and suitable clinical actions.

## 2.3 Communication of genetic test results

Depending on the institution and model used for testing and result disclosure, results may be communicated to a patient or parent/guardian by a medical provider (e.g., a specialty physician or nurse practitioner) or a genetic counselor. Only providers with sufficient knowledge in interpreting the genetic result and providing post-test counseling to patients should return the result. Otherwise, referral to a genetics professional is warranted. Results may be disclosed in an in-person setting, via video visit, or by telephone. Result disclosures are best done in a setting free from interruptions while providing opportunity for discussion and questions. The discussion should be conducted in a sensitive way, and the provider should watch or listen for clues of distress. It is important that sufficient silent time is allowed for the patient to absorb and reflect on the information provided. If the patient is not outwardly displaying a response to the results, targeted questions can be used to assess if they understood and how they feel about the information provided.

It is important that the following components of results disclosure are clearly communicated to patients and families:

1. The test result itself, including providing the patient with a copy of the result and explaining the nomenclature. For example, in the case of cardiogenomic multi-gene panel testing with a P/LP result, this means pointing out the gene with identified variant(s) and explaining the type of variant identified and how this is (likely) disease-causing.

2. The implications of this result. In the case of a negative or VUS result, for example, it may mean informing the patient that additional testing may be ordered in the future and that a negative result does not rule out the chance of having an underlying genetic etiology. In the case of a positive result, the patient should be informed of the relevance of the finding to their personal situation (e.g., does the result fully explain their phenotype?)

3. Any anticipated and/or guideline-indicated health care changes. There may be specialty clinics or specialty providers that can be discussed, or brief overviews of imaging or procedures that may be recommended and their anticipated frequency, or lifestyle changes that are indicated.

4. The implications for family members, including a discussion of inheritance patterns and cascade testing options. For example, if a condition is inherited in an autosomal dominant pattern with reduced penetrance and variable expressivity, this will need to be explained, as well as how family members can find out their variant status. Some genetic testing companies have time frames in which familial testing can be done at a reduced cost, which should be shared. Also, it's not uncommon for patients to be unaware that relatives who live far away can still benefit from genetic testing. The provider/counselor can be a resource for family members both in terms of connecting family members with providers/genetic counselors local to them and with arranging cascade testing.

5. The availability of resources and support services. After delivering a genetic result, it is important to check in with the patient and understand their needs. What questions or concerns do they have, and what credible informational

resources can you direct them to or provide? Do they have a support person at home, or perhaps they have an existing relationship with a therapist? There are resources that can be shared with patients, such as support groups or national foundations (e.g., the Dilated Cardiomyopathy Foundation, the Family Heart Foundation, the European Heart Network, etc.).

### 2.3.1 Communicating VUS results

Communicating VUS results to patients presents some additional challenges that warrant consideration. The terminology itself can sound confusing, and research has shown that, in some cases, a VUS can cause a higher level of concern for patients than a negative test result [15]. As aforementioned, ACMG/AMP (2015) guidelines state, "a variant of uncertain significance should not be used in clinical decision making.", and similarly, the Association for Clinical Genomic Science (ACGS) recommended (2016) the adoption of the ACMG guidelines in the UK [16]. According to the 2024 ACGS guidelines, "Variants of uncertain significance should generally only be considered for reporting where there is a high level of supporting evidence and additional evidence might be obtained to allow re-classification as (likely) pathogenic."

The Association for Clinical Genomic Science (ACGS) Best Practice Guidelines for Variant Classification in Rare Disease 2020 indicate situations when reporting a VUS on a test report would be inappropriate. These include (1.) instances when variants reported in peer-reviewed literature and databases subsequently were downgraded based on emerging scientific evidence, (2.) instances when the variant type or mechanism is a mismatch with the established disease mechanism, and (3.) instances when a VUS is identified in a gene associated with an autosomal recessive condition without a second variant being identified.

### 2.3.2 Communicating incidental findings or secondary findings

When clinical or research genetic testing is done, the test report may contain results unrelated to the indication for testing that are unexpected. The ACMG offers guidelines for returning actionable SFs; however, management of IFs remains a topic of debate [11, 17]. Laboratory consent forms may offer patients or parents/guardians the choice to opt in or out of receiving actionable SFs. Laboratories (or potentially, on a larger scale, professional societies) should have or should create guidelines regarding detecting and returning IFs. In situations where patients opt to receive results, the return of results process should include notifying the patient or parent/legal guardian, as well as the patient's relevant health care provider(s), and ensuring the result(s) is incorporated into the Electronic Medical Record [18]. Ideally, a genetic professional should be involved in this process. In cases of testing minors, guidelines need to be established as to what unsolicited information should be disclosed to balance the autonomy and interests of the child, as well as the parental rights and needs (not) to receive information that may be in the interest of their (future) family [19].

### 2.3.3 International recommendations for return of results

When returning results for clinical genomic sequencing, there are international recommendations in place to guide reporting. ACMG published its first version of recommendations for reporting incidental findings in clinical exome and genome sequencing in 2013, with version 3.2 released in August 2023, with a shift to using the term SFs in later versions to signify that the variants found in recommended genes are part of a pre-determined gene list and not "accidentally" identified [20–22]. Specifically, it states that SFs should be returned to patients and recommends reporting variants of specified classes or types in genes that have been carefully selected by the Working Group on Incidental Findings in Clinical Exome and Genome Sequencing. The number of genes on the list is updated annually. The ACMG SF v3.2 list consists of eighty-one genes.

These ACMG recommendations have been internationally impactful, motivating other countries to compile their own recommendations [19]. In 2013, the European Society of Human Genetics (ESHG) provided recommendations for health care professionals on the analysis, interpretation, and communication of diagnostic genetic testing [23]. The policy recommends using targeted genomics sequencing or analysis as a possible way to reduce unsolicited or uninterpretable findings. Additionally, filtering should be implemented to limit analysis to specific genes and those with clinical utility. A similar approach for returning results is suggested in Canada's 2015 policy [24]. The policy states that WES and WGS should be done only to interrogate sequence variation in genes known to cause disease and only after genetic counseling has been provided. They recommend a cautious approach to returning incidental findings and do not suggest the intentional clinical analysis of (medically actionable) disease-causing genes unrelated to the indication for testing. The Canadian College of Medical Genetics recommends using bioinformatic filtering specific to the testing indication to reduce discovery of IFs to reduce economic and emotional burden. Labs that do include assessment of IFs should ensure patients competent in decision-making are given the pre-test option to opt in or out of receiving these findings and should be informed of the type of IF that could occur. In minors, highly penetrant conditions that are medically actionable in childhood should be returned to parents, while results indicating risk for adult-onset conditions should only be returned if the parents request this and if disclosure could prevent serious health ramifications to the parent or a family member. The patient/family should receive genetic counseling following the return of the result.

It is important to note that recommendations and guidelines for returning genomic research results and IFs and SFs are quite variable and that efforts are underway to standardize them. Discrepancies can interfere with international research collaboration and, thus, scientific progress. For more information on the return of research results internationally, see [24].

### 2.3.4 Misattributed parentage

IFs and SFs are typically unexpected results. Another type of unexpected result that genetic testing may reveal is misattributed parentage, where genetic testing uncovers that either or both parents are genetically unrelated to a child. The most common form of misattributed parentage is non-paternity, a term referring to when the father is genetically unrelated to the child [25]. Misattributed parentage may be revealed when conducting cascade genetic testing, VUS-resolution family studies, or trio testing for WES or WGS, and is not uncommon. Reporting this information can lead to life-altering consequences for patients, and the literature lacks agreement as to whether it should be disclosed. Up to date, there are no clear guidelines or position statements to guide clinicians on the return of results involving misattributed parentage, although the American Society of Human Genetics (ASHG) does recommend that during pre-test genetic counseling patients (or parents/guardians) be educated that genetic testing can potentially reveal misattributed parentage. In 2015, a team of experts collaborated on an article in the *American Journal of Human Genetics* and stated that, "While honoring their broad responsibility to be truthful with patients and their families, we recommend that health care providers avoid disclosure of misattributed parentage unless there is a clear medical benefit that outweighs the potential harms" [25]. Similarly, a 2019 article in *Genetics in Medicine* states that "clinical relevance should determine whether or not to disclose results in the clinic" [26]. However, different views had also been previously expressed, such as the stance presented in The Lancet (2001), which states that clinicians should respect the autonomy of their patients and that withholding information on misattributed parentage undermines the rights of patients to make autonomous decisions. Withholding this information could lead patients and couples to make misinformed decisions [27]. The article characterizes the decision to withhold information on misattributed parentage as "unjustifiably paternalistic," implying that the clinician is exerting undue control over the disclosure process, indicating that the clinician assumes undue authority over what the patient or couple is permitted to know, thereby undermining patient autonomy, transparent communication, and informed decision-making.

When deciding whether to return such results, careful consideration must be given and the utmost care taken if disclosing misattributed parentage to patients. Importantly, determining how or whether to document instances of misattributed parentage in the medical records is essential to prevent accidental disclosure or unneeded investigation in the future [26]. A 2024 qualitative study explored the experiences of genetic counselors with non-paternity and found that when deciding whether or not to reveal non-paternity, genetic counselors balanced moral concepts of patient autonomy, the relevance of non-paternity to the medical scenario, and preventing harm [28]. Take, for example, the situation where a child is diagnosed with Jervell and Lange-Nielsen syndrome, an autosomal recessive form of long QT syndrome (LQTS). Suppose that trio genetic testing through WES reveals non-paternity, and the genetic provider is faced with whether or not to reveal this information. Withholding that non-paternity was discovered could leave the couple to understand that any of their future children have a 25% chance of also having Jervell and Lange-Nielsen syndrome, when in reality, the risk would be negligible. On the other hand, revealing the non-paternity could significantly impact the couple's relationship if the chance of identifying non-paternity was not previously discussed before genetic testing. This scenario highlights the importance of including a discussion of misattributed parentage/non-paternity during pre-testing genetic counseling.

## 2.4 Risk determination for family members/cascade testing

Once a genetic diagnosis is made in the proband, the risk of other family members' needs to be calculated, taking into consideration the inheritance pattern. For example, in autosomal dominant conditions, each first-degree relative has a 50% chance of carrying the variant, with potential variability in phenotypic severity (due to variable expressivity) and age of onset, as well as the possibility of asymptomatic carriers due to reduced penetrance. In autosomal recessive conditions, both parents must be carriers, giving each of their offsprings a 25% risk of being affected and a 50% chance of being carriers. For X-linked recessive conditions, XY offspring of carrier mothers have a 50% risk of being affected, while XX offspring have a 50% chance of being carriers. Therefore, knowledge of the disease-causing variant can help guide further testing, clinical surveillance, therapeutic strategy choices, and family planning of the carriers.

Furthermore, for family members at risk, cascade testing is indicated. The cascade testing process starts with first-degree relatives (parents, siblings, children) of index cases (i.e., the family member in whom a disease-causing variant was identified) and then proceeds to second- (grandparents/grandchildren, aunts/uncles, nieces/nephews, half-siblings) and third-degree relatives (great-grandparents/great-grand-children, first cousins). The detection of the disease-causing variant in asymptomatic relatives will guide downstream medical decisions, including prevention measures and clinical surveillance strategies. On the other hand, relatives found not to carry the disease-causing variant do not require further clinical workup. It is noted, however, as discussed in Section 2.5, that careful consideration is needed when family members are asymptomatic children or adolescents [29].

Ultimately, a genetic diagnosis in the proband shifts risk assessment from an individual concern to a pro-active family-wide strategy, enabling comprehensive and cost-effective management of cardiovascular genetic conditions [30].

## 2.5 Testing minors

Genetic testing is indicated when a person presents with a phenotype associated with a cardiovascular genetic condition, regardless of age. However, when testing minors, a vulnerable population unable to provide consent, a specific set of considerations must be addressed. The American Academy of Pediatrics (AAP) and the American College of Medical Genetics and Genomics (ACMG) established guidelines in 2013 recommending that genetic diagnostic testing in minors should follow the same standards as other medical diagnostic procedures, necessitating full informed consent [31]. Carrier testing should generally be avoided unless the results have immediate health implications for the minor or if the minor is actively considering reproduction. Predictive genetic testing for adult-onset disorders is also discouraged, except in specific cases where it is clinically justified and only if accompanied by genetic counseling. In the 2020 statement of the American Heart Association on genetic testing for inherited cardiovascular diseases, it is stated that in minors a well-defined cardiovascular genetic phenotype must be present before considering genetic testing [32]. A family-centered approach involving pre- and post-test counseling is crucial. While parental or guardian consent is typically obtained, the child's assent should be considered to respect their autonomy. Discussions should clarify the benefits, limitations, and potential outcomes of genetic testing, ensuring both parents and children understand the implications. The psychological impact of test results on minors and their families must be managed carefully, including addressing any anxiety related to outcomes and future health.

Genetic testing for minors who are unaffected but at risk given a known molecular diagnosis in the family should also be approached with caution. Multiple international position statements and professional guidelines discourage predictive genetic testing for adult-onset genetic conditions for individuals under age eighteen when results will not alter childhood medical management or be of substantial benefit. This provides individuals with the autonomy, as they reach adulthood, to decide on genetic testing for themselves. Due to this recommendation, it is less typical for genetic testing for adult-onset cardiac conditions to be conducted in minors. However, for patient- or family-specific reasons or individual requests, genetic testing in minors for adult-onset conditions does occur in multiple countries [33]. Research has been done and more is underway that involves parents and minors to understand their preference regarding learning of LP/P variants for adult-onset conditions in children. Results have indicated a preference to receive results for actionable variants for the purposes of awareness, proactiveness, and control over their child's health, while some studies have indicated reservations about learning of variants in children related to untreatable adult-onset conditions [34, 35]. In general, if results for adult-onset conditions are being returned to minors, shared decision-making between the provider/genetic counselor and parents/guardians should be carried out to determine when the child is ready to learn the results and what resources may be helpful in supporting them. This is largely because of differing levels of maturity in children, personality traits, and mental health states.

In most cases, however, testing should be deferred until the child can participate in the decision-making process, unless a clear medical benefit justifies early testing, such as an intervention to prevent disease onset or reduce morbidity. Reduced penetrance and variable expressivity, characteristic of cardiovascular genetic disorders, introduce uncertainty, as a positive result cannot predict if, when, or how the disease may manifest. In such situations, understanding the average age of onset of the disorder in question and the family's disease presentation can guide the appropriateness of testing. If a child tests positive, regular follow-up—such as annual evaluations—is recommended. While this surveillance can be life-saving, initiating it too early may lead to unnecessary costs and anxiety. Counseling should address these concerns.

Familial hypercholesterolemia (FH) genetic testing guidelines [36], on the other hand, highlight the importance of early identification and management to mitigate the risk of premature atherosclerotic cardiovascular disease in children. Children with a strong clinical suspicion of FH—evidenced by elevated LDLc levels and a relevant family history—should be offered genetic testing. The AAP also recommends universal lipid screening for children aged 9–11, and as early as 2 years for those with a family history of FH (Expert Panel on Integrated Guidelines for Cardiovascular Health and Risk Reduction in Children and Adolescents & National Heart, Lung, and Blood Institute, 2011). Genetic testing in unaffected at-risk children is recommended, as FH hyperlipidemia is present from birth, leading to chronic exposure of LDLc and associated CAD risk if untreated.

When the child has the capacity to understand the meaning of the result, at some level, the results for the pediatric-onset condition should be delivered in an age-appropriate manner to the child in the presence of a parent or guardian. This would best be done via in-person consultation or potentially via video visit. For children too young to understand the meaning of the result, or in situations where a minor has an underlying cognitive, emotional, or psychological condition, the parent or guardian should be provided with the result and counseling. When the child is of an appropriate age and maturity level and has the capacity to understand the meaning of the result, they should be offered genetic counseling.

## 2.6 Psychosocial implications of CVD genetic testing/supporting patients and their families

Being diagnosed with a cardiovascular condition and undergoing genetic testing can cause different psychological responses. These responses will be impacted by the timeline in which they occur. For example, did a clinical diagnosis come before genetic testing? Did genetic testing reveal previously unknown increased risk for CVD in the absence of a phenotype or family history (as in cases of SFs or population screening)? Last, was genetic testing done in the context of a known personal or family history of CVD? Research has shown that health-related quality of life is negatively impacted by a medical diagnosis and the severity of that phenotype, activity restrictions, and side effects from needed medications [37]. The addition of genetic testing after a clinical diagnosis may positively or negatively impact pre-existing psychological issues.

The literature is somewhat split regarding the psychosocial impact of CVD genetic testing on patients with an identified disease-causing variant, with some feeling empowered by the knowledge and relief from the uncertainty of not knowing, while others experienced increased worry and fear. Wynn et al. found that those who received a P/LP genetic test result were more negatively impacted (in terms of uncertainty and distress) than those who received a B/LB result [38]. Those with a VUS were more negatively impacted than those with B/LB results, but not as negatively impacted as those with P/LP results. Oliveri et al. performed a systematic review of the psychological implications of genetic testing reported in nine studies that evaluated the impact of genetic testing related to different cardiovascular clinical conditions, including LQTS, thrombophilia, cardiomyopathy, arterial hypertension, and FH [39]. Generally, similar scales were used to assess the quality of life and risk perception for assessing the psychological implications of genetic testing in these studies. Somewhat contrary to the findings of Wynn et al. [38] and Oliveri et al. [39] reported that these studies found no post-testing negative impacts on quality of life or substantial increase in distress or anxiety. Similarly, a study by Hickey et al. [15] that assessed the impact of genetic testing for cardiac arrhythmias found that positive genetic results did not negatively impact patient well-being. The context in which genetic testing is done will influence patients' responses to CVD genetic testing results.

### 2.6.1 Phenotype-positive individuals

In many instances, positive genetic testing in phenotype-positive individuals does not alter diagnosis, prognosis, or management. In such cases, genetic testing rarely increases anxiety and worry. However, genetic testing in individuals who have certain variants in genes related to hypertrophic cardiomyopathy (HCM), dilated cardiomyopathy, arrhythmogenic right ventricular cardiomyopathy, LQTS, Marfan syndrome, aortopathies, and FH can impact diagnosis, prognosis, and management and therefore may impact levels of anxiety [40]. Possible negative impacts of CVD genetic testing on individuals with a CVD phenotype include doubt of their diagnosis if testing is negative or frustration that a cause remains unidentified [40]. Additionally, patients who are found to have a VUS are left with uncertainty regarding the meaning of their result, which can produce a variety of responses, including worry, disappointment, frustration, regret, relief, and anticipation for reclassification [41]. Possible positive impacts of CVD genetic testing on individuals with a known phenotype may include strengthened confidence in a given diagnosis, improved adherence with management recommendations, and relief at having a result that can lead to informative testing for family members [40, 42].

### 2.6.2 Phenotype-negative individuals

For un- or pre-symptomatic individuals who test negative for a familial variant, genetic testing often offers reassurance and, potentially, relief. However, some of those who test negative may also experience survivor guilt that other family members have inherited a familial variant that they did not.

In the same context, but where a familial variant is identified in an individual, there can be both positive and negative impacts of CVD genetic testing. Positive impacts may include relieving uncertainty about their genotype status, providing adjustment time, and the ability to inform life planning. It can also promote a sense of control, allowing individuals to be pro-active in health care and behavioral choices [40]. Conversely, negative implications of genetic testing may include heightened anxiety related to genotype-associated risks and concerns over transmitting these variants to children and other relatives, altered self-perception, and fears of discrimination or how the results might influence significant life decisions [40]. Positive genetic testing on un- or pre-symptomatic individuals can also lead to frustration or confusion. One study reported that individuals who tested positive for a CVD-associated genetic variant while lacking clinical symptoms expressed skepticism about the value of such testing, particularly for minors. This uncertainty stemmed from concerns about the implications of modifying a child's behavior and imposing restrictions based on a genetic predisposition for a condition that has not yet manifested [43].

Some individuals are more likely to experience a negative psychological impact after having genetic testing, including those with a history of depression or anxiety and those whose subjective perception of risk associated with the condition before result disclosure is in conflict with the actual genetic test result [43, 44].

It is well established that uncertainty regarding health risks impacts coping and adaptation. Uncertainty regarding symptoms and risk associated with a CVD genotype can negatively impact psychological well-being and quality of life [45, 46]. Levels of uncertainty may vary depending on the phenotype associated with the CVD variant identified in an individual. For example, even though many individuals with HCM have a relatively benign experience, they may face a level of uncertainty that is real, but by comparison, less than in individuals who have a variant that substantially impacts mortality risk [47]. Additionally, the ability to adapt to a diagnosis or risk of a future diagnosis can vary and may depend on pre-existing mental status and individual intrinsic components such as a search for meaning and motivation to regain control and restore self-esteem [48]. Given the multitude of factors influencing patients' reactions to genetic testing outcomes, a personalized approach to genetic counseling is essential.

### 2.6.3 Supporting adaptation

Providing pre-test genetic counseling to patients, as described in the chapter "Genetic Counseling for Cardiovascular Disease—Part A: Pre-test approaches & considerations" of this book, can be the first step to helping them adapt to receiving results during post-test genetic counseling. Some genetic counselors use the models of motivational interviewing (MI) and shared decision-making (SDM) to support patient-centered care during both pre-test and post-test genetic counseling to ensure decisions are being made that align with personal values and desires, which may facilitate later adjustment. In the post-test context in particular, MI and SDM are critical, particularly when communicating complex or uncertain results. After test results are available, these strategies help in addressing patients' emotional responses, guiding discussions on the implications of results for medical management, and formulating a plan that incorporates the patient's preferences and goals. MI is particularly useful in supporting patients who may need to make lifestyle or behavioral changes based on their genetic results, while SDM ensures that subsequent medical decisions, such as surveillance or family testing, are made collaboratively. Rollnick et al. describe the step-by-step process of motivational interviewing, which requires the provider to "engage with and work in collaboration with patients, emphasize their autonomy over decision-making, and elicit their motivation for change" [49]. Motivational interviewing can be helpful when patients have not been engaged with their health-care and have not taken action to understand genetic risk or adhere to management recommendations. In SDM, providers help patients to understand their options and make informed choices [50]. This occurs when providers share knowledge about the scenario at hand, collaborate with patients, and help to elicit patient perspectives and preferences. The hope is that the final decision aligns with patient values. SDM can be very helpful when genetic counselors are discussing genetic testing and the steps or actions patients can take after results disclosure. Details on the process of shared decision-making can be found in Stiggelbout et al. [51].

Research has shown that psychological distress following CVD genetic testing is generally low [39, 44]. However, in those who experience increased anxiety and distress, psychological well-being can be improved in those with a genetic condition or known increased risk with clinical or psychological interventions [48]. Genetics professionals can assist with adaptation to a risk or genetic condition [48, 52]. Biesecker and Erby [48] suggest that in the course of the genetics consultation, the genetics professional can help the patients strategize the controllable aspects of their condition, such as how to discuss it with others and make a treatment and manage-ment plan. They can also help the patient or parent to recognize personal successes of managing medical-related stress and determine if the past strategies can be used in the current scenario. Additionally, in taking personal and family histories, genetics professionals typically learn of underlying anxiety and depression. Since we know these conditions pose a greater risk of an unfavorable psychosocial impact following genetic testing, providers can be prepared to provide needed assistance and support to these individuals, including being ready to refer patients for targeted therapy [44].

Another strategy to support adaptation is allowing enough time during patient vis-its for discussion, questions, and education. It has been demonstrated that educating patients about their condition to promote understanding can be effective at relieving their concerns and helping them to adapt [46]. For example, one study found that in patients with HCM, the information that was provided to them, the time providers spent with the patient and the staff-patient relationship, and patient understanding of the condition were related to the patient's psychological well-being, adjustment, worry, and compliance with management [47]. Managing patients with HCM and their families with a multidisciplinary approach that includes genetic counseling is beneficial, and further, having patients attend CVD-specific genetics clinics may positively impact adjustment and levels of worry [47].

In the context of unaffected individuals learning about increased risk for cancer based on genetic testing (that could be applied to the CVD context), Dean and Davidson found four strategies that could help patients manage the medical uncer-tainty [53]. These strategies include seeking health care providers (1) as informational sources, (2) as partners for decision-making, (3) as a resource for supportive com-munication, and (4) seeking referrals for social support networks. Further, their research showed that providers who are knowledgeable and can provide information and answers to patient questions, who verify patient understanding, and who pro-vide helpful resources help manage uncertainty by highlighting options and helping patients ascribe meaning.

Genetic counselors can validate any feelings the patients discuss while being prepared to refer and provide appropriate resources. There are licensed therapists or psychologists who specialize in chronic health conditions, genetics, or medical decision-making who may be able to help families weigh their concerns or sociocultural morals and feelings against the information that genetic testing provides. For example, some families struggle with a decision about predictive testing for a minor or may have intrusive thoughts after the sudden loss of a loved one. Genetic counselors should be able to identify pathology and scope of practice limitations and refer to other professionals who can provide longer-term specialized care. Patient support and advocacy organizations often have information modules, phone numbers, and emails available so patients can receive further support and information. Condition-specific foundations, advocacy organizations, and support groups can help families as they undergo genetic testing and, in some cases, provide relatable experiences and emotional support. For example, the Sudden Arrhythmia Death Syndrome Foundation (SADS) provides information on genetic testing, support groups for individuals with different forms of arrhythmias, educational events, and a family registry that can help families connect with relevant clinical trials. Similarly, the DCM Foundation has an impressive list of DCM-specific and gene-specific online support groups that patients can access as they navigate genetic testing decisions and potentially seek support following a genetic diagnosis.

Furthermore, family sharing letters can be provided to patients to help with family communication. For children, there are books available that discuss in age-appropriate ways when a parent has a certain genetic condition. Genetic counselors can also facilitate the presence of a support person during consultations, particularly when patients exhibit signs of distress or emotional discomfort. This approach ensures a supportive environment and promotes effective communication, allowing patients to process complex genetic information with the help of someone they trust.

## 3. Conclusions

In conclusion, the rapidly evolving field of cardiovascular disease (CVD) genetics holds tremendous promise for improving the prevention, diagnosis, and management of at-risk individuals and families. As the use of genetic testing in CVD becomes more widespread, the role of specialized genetic counseling is increasingly critical in supporting patients and clinicians throughout the entire genetic testing process [54]. The post-testing phase is essential for ensuring that complex genetic information is accurately interpreted, incidental findings are managed appropriately, and challenging situations, such as non-paternity disclosure or testing minors, are handled with sensitivity and care. Genetic counselors play a central role in guiding healthcare providers and patients through these complexities, ensuring that test results are integrated meaningfully into patient care and family risk management strategies. The expanding use of tools and databases for variant interpretation, along with the growing emphasis on family risk assessment through cascade testing, presents new opportunities for early intervention and targeted management. However, these advances also highlight the need for ongoing education, interdisciplinary collaboration, and adherence to ethical guidelines. As the field continues to evolve, close collaboration between cardiologists and genetic counselors will be essential to delivering personalized, genetically informed care that empowers patients and optimizes health outcomes for families affected by cardiovascular disease.

## Acknowledgements

DS was supported by CUREPLaN, a grant from the Leducq Foundation for Cardiovascular Research (18CVD01).

## Conflict of interest

The authors declare no conflict of interest.

## Author details

Despina Sanoudou[1*], Jessica Goehringer[2,3] and Ana Morales[2,4]

1 Clinical Genomics and Pharmacogenomics Unit, 4th Department of Internal Medicine, "Attikon" Hospital, Medical School, National and Kapodistrian University of Athens, Athens, Greece

2 Geisinger, Danville, PA, USA

3 Geisinger College of Health Sciences, Scranton, PA, USA

4 Translational Health Sciences Program, School of Medicine and Health Sciences, The George Washington University, District of Columbia, USA

*Address all correspondence to: dsanoudou@med.uoa.gr

**IntechOpen**

# References

[1] Richards S, Aziz N, Bale S, Bick D, Das S, Gastier-Foster J, et al. Standards and guidelines for the interpretation of sequence variants: A joint consensus recommendation of the American College of Medical Genetics and Genomics and the Association for Molecular Pathology. Genetics in Medicine. 2015;**17**(5):405-424

[2] McCormick EM, Lott MT, Dulik MC, Shen L, Attimonelli M, Vitale O, et al. Specifications of the ACMG/AMP standards and guidelines for mitochondrial DNA variant interpretation. Human Mutation. 2020;**41**(12):2028-2057

[3] Riggs ER, Andersen EF, Cherry AM, Kantarci S, Kearney H, Patel A, et al. Technical standards for the interpretation and reporting of constitutional copy-number variants: A joint consensus recommendation of the American College of Medical Genetics and Genomics (ACMG) and the clinical genome resource (ClinGen). Genetics in Medicine. 2020;**22**(2):245-257

[4] Boggan RM, Lim A, Taylor RW, McFarland R, Pickett SJ. Resolving complexity in mitochondrial disease: Towards precision medicine. Molecular Genetics and Metabolism. 2019;**128**(1-2):19-29

[5] Mates J, Mademont-Soler I, Del Olmo B, Ferrer-Costa C, Coll M, Perez-Serra A, et al. Role of copy number variants in sudden cardiac death and related diseases: Genetic analysis and translation into clinical practice. European Journal of Human Genetics: EJHG. 2018;**26**(7):1014-1025

[6] Singer ES, Ross SB, Skinner JR, Weintraub RG, Ingles J, Semsarian C, et al. Characterization of clinically relevant copy-number variants from exomes of patients with inherited heart disease and unexplained sudden cardiac death. Genetics in Medicine. 2021;**23**(1):86-93

[7] Chen E, Facio FM, Aradhya KW, Rojahn S, Hatchell KE, Aguilar S, et al. Rates and classification of variants of uncertain significance in hereditary disease genetic testing. JAMA Network Open. 2023;**6**(10):e2339571

[8] Costa S, Medeiros-Domingo A, Gasperetti A, Akdis D, Berger W, James CA, et al. Impact of genetic variant reassessment on the diagnosis of arrhythmogenic right ventricular cardiomyopathy based on the 2010 task force criteria. Circulation Genomic and Precision Medicine. 2021;**14**(1):e003047

[9] Mersch J, Brown N, Pirzadeh-Miller S, Mundt E, Cox HC, Brown K, et al. Prevalence of variant reclassification following hereditary cancer genetic testing. Journal of the American Medical Association. 2018;**320**(12):1266-1274

[10] Gudmundsson S, Singer-Berk M, Watts NA, Phu W, Goodrich JK, Solomonson M, et al. Variant interpretation using population databases: Lessons from gnomAD. Human Mutation. 2022;**43**(8): 1012-1030

[11] Bowling KM, Thompson ML, Kelly MA, Scollon S, Slavotinek AM, Powell BC, et al. Return of non-ACMG recommended incidental genetic findings to pediatric patients: Considerations and opportunities from experiences in genomic sequencing. Genome Medicine. 2022;**14**(1):131

[12] Schwartz MLB, McCormick CZ, Lazzeri AL, Lindbuchler DM, Hallquist MLG, Manickam K, et al. A model for genome-first care: Returning secondary genomic findings to participants and their healthcare providers in a large research cohort. American Journal of Human Genetics. 2018;**103**(3):328-337

[13] Elfatih A, Mohammed I, Abdelrahman D, Mifsud B. Frequency and management of medically actionable incidental findings from genome and exome sequencing data: A systematic review. Physiological Genomics. 2021;**53**(9):373-384

[14] eMERGE Clinical Annotation Working Group. Frequency of genomic secondary findings among 21,915 eMERGE network participants. Genetics in Medicine. 2020;**22**(9):1470-1477

[15] Mighton C, Shickh S, Uleryk E, Pechlivanoglou P, Bombard Y. Clinical and psychological outcomes of receiving a variant of uncertain significance from multigene panel testing or genomic sequencing: A systematic review and meta-analysis. Genetics in Medicine. 2021;**23**(1):22-33

[16] Sian Ellard ELB et al. ACGS Best Practice Guidelines for Variant Classification in Rare Disease 2020. London, UK: Association for Clinical Genomic Science; 2020

[17] van der Schoot V, Haer-Wigman L, Feenstra I, Tammer F, Oerlemans AJM, van Koolwijk MPA, et al. Lessons learned from unsolicited findings in clinical exome sequencing of 16,482 individuals. European Journal of Human Genetics: EJHG. 2022;**30**(2):170-177

[18] Wiesner GL, Kulchak Rahm A, Appelbaum P, Aufox S, Bland ST, Blout CL, et al. Returning results in the genomic era: Initial experiences of the eMERGE network. Journal of Personalized Medicine. 2020;**10**(2):1-12

[19] Saelaert M, Mertes H, De Baere E, Devisch I. Incidental or secondary findings: An integrative and patient-inclusive approach to the current debate. European Journal of Human Genetics: EJHG. 2018;**26**(10):1424-1431

[20] ACMG Board of Directors. ACMG policy statement: Updated recommendations regarding analysis and reporting of secondary findings in clinical genome-scale sequencing. Genetics in Medicine. 2015;**17**(1):68-69

[21] Green RC, Berg JS, Grody WW, Kalia SS, Korf BR, Martin CL, et al. ACMG recommendations for reporting of incidental findings in clinical exome and genome sequencing. Genetics in Medicine. 2013;**15**(7):565-574

[22] Miller DT, Lee K, Abul-Husn NS, Amendola LM, Brothers K, Chung WK, et al. ACMG SF v3.2 list for reporting of secondary findings in clinical exome and genome sequencing: A policy statement of the American College of Medical Genetics and Genomics (ACMG). Genetics in Medicine. 2023;**25**(8):100866

[23] van El CG, Cornel MC, Borry P, Hastings RJ, Fellmann F, Hodgson SV, et al. Whole-genome sequencing in health care: Recommendations of the European Society of Human Genetics. European Journal of Human Genetics: EJHG. 2013;**21**(6):580-584

[24] Thorogood A, Dalpe G, Knoppers BM. Return of individual genomic research results: Are laws and policies keeping step? European Journal of Human Genetics: EJHG. 2019;**27**(4):535-546

[25] Botkin JR, Belmont JW, Berg JS, Berkman BE, Bombard Y, Holm IA, et al. Points to consider: Ethical, legal, and psychosocial implications of genetic testing in children and adolescents. American Journal of Human Genetics. 2015;**97**(1):6-21

[26] Wright CF, Parker M, Lucassen AM. When genomic medicine reveals misattributed genetic relationships-the debate about disclosure revisited. Genetics in Medicine. 2019;**21**(1):97-101

[27] Lucassen A, Parker M. Revealing false paternity: Some ethical considerations. Lancet. 2001;**357**(9261):1033-1035

[28] Cunningham E, Hays S, Wainstein T, Zierhut H, Virani A, Tryon R. Exploring genetic counselors' experiences with non-paternity in clinical settings. Journal of Genetic Counseling. 2024:1-13

[29] Ingles J, McGaughran J, Scuffham PA, Atherton J, Semsarian C. A cost-effectiveness model of genetic testing for the evaluation of families with hypertrophic cardiomyopathy. Heart. 2012;**98**(8):625-630

[30] Catchpool M, Ramchand J, Martyn M, Hare DL, James PA, Trainer AH, et al. A cost-effectiveness model of genetic testing and periodical clinical screening for the evaluation of families with dilated cardiomyopathy. Genetics in Medicine. 2019;**21**(12):2815-2822

[31] Clayton EW. How much control do children and adolescents have over genomic testing, parental access to their results, and parental communication of those results to others? The Journal of Law, Medicine & Ethics: A Journal of the American Society of Law, Medicine & Ethics. 2015;**43**(3):538-544

[32] Musunuru K, Hershberger RE, Day SM, Klinedinst NJ, Landstrom AP, Parikh VN, et al. Genetic testing for inherited cardiovascular diseases: A scientific statement from the American Heart Association. Circulation Genomic and Precision Medicine. 2020;**13**(4):e000067

[33] Fenwick A, Plantinga M, Dheensa S, Lucassen A. Predictive genetic testing of children for adult-onset conditions: Negotiating requests with parents. Journal of Genetic Counseling. 2017;**26**(2):244-250

[34] Sapp JC, Dong D, Stark C, Ivey LE, Hooker G, Biesecker LG, et al. Parental attitudes, values, and beliefs toward the return of results from exome sequencing in children. Clinical Genetics. 2014;**85**(2):120-126

[35] Savatt JM, Wagner JK, Joffe S, Rahm AK, Williams MS, Bradbury AR, et al. Pediatric reporting of genomic results study (PROGRESS): A mixed-methods, longitudinal, observational cohort study protocol to explore disclosure of actionable adult- and pediatric-onset genomic variants to minors and their parents. BMC Pediatrics. 2020;**20**(1):222

[36] Sturm AC, Knowles JW, Gidding SS, Ahmad ZS, Ahmed CD, Ballantyne CM, et al.; Convened by the Familial Hypercholesterolemia Foundation. Clinical genetic testing for familial hypercholesterolemia: JACC scientific expert panel. Journal of the American College of Cardiology. 7 Aug 2018;**72**(6):662-680. DOI: 10.1016/j.jacc.2018.05.044

[37] Cox S, O'Donoghue AC, McKenna WJ, Steptoe A. Health related quality of life and psychological wellbeing in patients with

hypertrophic cardiomyopathy. Heart. 1997;**78**(2):182-187

[38] Wynn J, Holland DT, Duong J, Ahimaz P, Chung WK. Examining the psychosocial impact of genetic testing for cardiomyopathies. Journal of Genetic Counseling. 2018;**27**(4):927-934

[39] Oliveri S, Ferrari F, Manfrinati A, Pravettoni G. A systematic review of the psychological implications of genetic testing: A comparative analysis among cardiovascular, neurodegenerative and cancer diseases. Frontiers in Genetics. 2018;**9**:624

[40] Aatre RD, Day SM. Psychological issues in genetic testing for inherited cardiovascular diseases. Circulation Cardiovascular Genetics. 2011;**4**(1):81-90

[41] Clift K, Macklin S, Halverson C, McCormick JB, Abu Dabrh AM, Hines S. Patients' views on variants of uncertain significance across indications. Journal of Community Genetics. 2020;**11**(2):139-145

[42] Marteau T, Senior V, Humphries SE, Bobrow M, Cranston T, Crook MA, et al. Psychological impact of genetic testing for familial hypercholesterolemia within a previously aware population: A randomized controlled trial. American Journal of Medical Genetics Part A. 2004;**128A**(3):285-293

[43] Ormondroyd E, Oates S, Parker M, Blair E, Watkins H. Pre-symptomatic genetic testing for inherited cardiac conditions: A qualitative exploration of psychosocial and ethical implications. European Journal of Human Genetics: EJHG. 2014;**22**(1):88-93

[44] Bordet C, Brice S, Maupain C, Gandjbakhch E, Isidor B, Palmyre A, et al. Psychosocial impact of predictive genetic testing in hereditary heart diseases: The PREDICT study. Journal of Clinical Medicine. 2020;**9**(5):1-14

[45] Carroll DL, Hamilton GA, McGovern BA. Changes in health status and quality of life and the impact of uncertainty in patients who survive life-threatening arrhythmias. Heart & Lung: The Journal of Critical Care. 1999;**28**(4):251-260

[46] Shiloh S, Avdor O, Goodman RM. Satisfaction with genetic counseling: Dimensions and measurement. American Journal of Medical Genetics. 1990;**37**(4):522-529

[47] Ingles J, Lind JM, Phongsavan P, Semsarian C. Psychosocial impact of specialized cardiac genetic clinics for hypertrophic cardiomyopathy. Genetics in Medicine. 2008;**10**(2):117-120

[48] Biesecker BB, Erby L. Adaptation to living with a genetic condition or risk: A mini-review. Clinical Genetics. Nov 2008;**74**(5):401-407. DOI: 10.1111/j.1399-0004.2008.01088.x

[49] Rollnick S, Butler CC, Kinnersley P, Gregory J, Mash B. Motivational Interviewing. BMJ. 2010;**340**:c1900

[50] Elwyn G, Dehlendorf C, Epstein RM, Marrin K, White J, Frosch DL. Shared decision making and motivational interviewing: Achieving patient-centered care across the spectrum of health care problems. Annals of Family Medicine. 2014;**12**(3):270-275

[51] Stiggelbout AM, Pieterse AH, De Haes JC. Shared decision making: Concepts, evidence, and practice. Patient Education and Counseling. 2015;**98**(10):1172-1179

[52] National Society of Genetic Counselors' Definition Task F, Resta R, Biesecker BB, Bennett RL, Blum S,

Hahn SE, et al. A new definition of genetic counseling: National Society of genetic counselors' task force report. Journal of Genetic Counseling. 2006;**15**(2):77-83

[53] Dean M, Davidson LG. Previvors' uncertainty management strategies for hereditary breast and ovarian cancer. Health Communication. 2018;**33**(2):122-130

[54] Morales A, Goehringer J, Sanoudou D. Evolving cardiovascular genetic counseling needs in the era of precision medicine. Frontiers in Cardiovascular Medicine. 2023;**10**:1161029